Radiology Interv

Questions for ST Radiology Intervie

Edited by

James Russell BSc MBChB MRCS PGCert

Radiology Registrar, Royal Free Hospital, London

Matthew Seager BSc MBChB MRCS

Radiology Registrar, St George's Hospital, London

© 2017 MD+ Publishing

All rights reserved. No part of this publication may be reproduced, stored in a retrieval system or transmitted in any form or by any means, electronic, mechanical, photocopying, recording or otherwise without the prior permission of the publisher or in accordance with the provisions of the Copyright, Designs and Patents Act 1988 or under the terms of any licence permitting limited copying issued by the Copyright Licensing Agency.

Published by: MD+ Publishing

Cover Design: Alexander Logan

ISBN-10: 0995662614

ISBN-13: 978-0-995662612

Printed in the United Kingdom

CONTENTS

Chapter 1. The Basics

1.1 Radiology in the UK 8
1.2 Radiology training 13
1.3 The ST1 application overview 17
1.4 The ST1 interview overview 20
1.5 The radiological CV 24
1.6 Interview technique 32

Chapter 2. The SRA

2.1 Introduction to the SRA 42
2.2 Professional Dilemmas *(PD/SJT)* 43
2.3 Clinical Problem Solving *(CPS)* 50

Chapter 3. Portfolio Station

3.1 Specific questions 60
   3.1.1 Clinical radiology experience 60
   3.1.2 Audit 62
   3.1.3 Teaching 64
   3.1.4 Exams 66
   3.1.5 Research 67

3.2 Motivational questions 69
   3.2.1 What is your proudest achievement? . . . 69
   3.2.2 What is your greatest strength? 70
   3.2.3 What is your main weakness? 71

3.3 Situational ability questions 74
   3.3.1 Communication skills 74
   3.3.2 Risk management 75
   3.3.3 Problem Solving 77
   3.3.4 Empathy 78
   3.3.5 Team work 80
   3.3.6 Time management 81
   3.3.7 Judgment 82
   3.3.8 Leadership 83

3.3.9 Conflict resolution. 85
3.3.10 Probity 86

Chapter 4. Commitment to Specialty Station

4.1 What are the greatest challenges facing radiology? 90
4.2 What do you think the future of radiology is? . 91
4.3 How will 7-day working affect radiology? . . . 92
4.4 How do radiologists learn from their mistakes? 93
4.5 What are the different subspecialties within radiology? 94
4.6 Tell us about radiology training 95
4.7 What is your preferred type of training scheme? 97
4.8 What is the role of the consultant radiologist? . 98
4.9 What can you bring to radiology? 99
4.10 What will you miss as a radiologist? 100
4.11 What is PACS? 101
4.12 What do you think of skills mix? 102
4.13 What are the harmful effects of ionising radiation? 103
4.14 What do you know about ionising radiation legislation in the UK? 104
4.15 What do you think of outsourcing? 105

Chapter 5. The Old Interview Stations

5.1 Report critique 107
5.2 Ethical scenarios 115
   5.2.1 Difficult procedure. 115
   5.2.2 Drunk colleague 117
   5.2.3 Scanning in pregnancy 119
   5.2.4 Confidentiality 121
   5.2.5 Radiation protection incident 124
   5.2.6 Contrast reaction 126
   5.2.7 Jehovah's Witness 128
   5.2.8 Inappropriate referral 130

Contributors

Many thanks to the following trainees and consultants who contributed to the text:

Anmol Malhotra BSc MBBS MRCP FRCR
Consultant radiologist, Royal Free Hospital, London

Vruti Dattani MA MBBS
Radiology registrar, Royal Free Hospital, London

Fern Adams MA (Cantab) MBBChir RAF
Radiology registrar, Royal Free Hospital, London

Geoffrey Chow BSc MBBS
Radiology registrar, Royal Free Hospital, London

Thomas Armstrong MBBS
Radiology registrar, Royal Free Hospital, London

Thomas Glover BA MA (Cantab) MBBChir
Radiology registrar, Chelsea and Westminster Hospital, London

Archie Keeling MBChB
Radiology registrar, Kings College Hospital, London

Mariam Jacob MBBS
Radiology registrar, University Hospitals of Leicester NHS Trust

Emily Ashworth MBBS MRCPCH
Radiology registrar, St George's Hospital, London

Thomas Welsh BSc MBChB
Radiology registrar, Peninsula Radiology Academy

Sara Ffrench-Constant BA (Oxon) MBBS
Radiology registrar, Imperial College Healthcare NHS Trust, London

Jay Jadeja BSc MBChB PGDip Medical Ultrasound
Frimley Health NHS Foundation Trust

Preface

Firstly, well done for picking radiology!

Medical imaging has become an essential part of safe and effective patient management and it just so follows that a radiology training post is one of the most sought-after training positions in the UK. This was reflected in the competition ratio in 2017, with around 1000 applicants competing for just over 260 posts. Those applying are from lots of different medical and surgical backgrounds, from FY2s to senior trainees across a variety of specialities. With this in mind we have created the following resource which aims to provide a comprehensive and balanced view of the current recruitment process and provide tips on how you can navigate the process to achieve your number one choice.

Written by high-scoring candidates at previous radiology interviews, this book features a large number of practice questions which have been asked in recent years. These will cover the preparation, portfolio and commitment to specialty stations which formed the basis of the 2017 interview. We recognise that the interview format has changed multiple times in recent years, and we have included a specific chapter on the old interview stations to ensure that your preparation is thorough and covers all the bases. The content is based on questions faced by candidates who have sat the three most recent interviews and we feel is representative of what you should expect be asked. Despite our best efforts, the interview format may still be subject to change but the broad themes covered should remain the same.

We hope this book will appeal to all those applying to radiology, regardless of grade or speciality.

We hope you enjoy and wish you luck in your applications.

James and Matt

1 THE BASICS

1.1 Radiology in the UK 8
1.2 Radiology training 13
1.3 The ST1 application overview 17
1.4 The ST1 interview overview 20
1.5 The radiological CV 24
1.6 Interview technique 32

1.1 Radiology in the UK

Medical imaging is used to diagnose, monitor and treat a multitude of diseases and is now at the very heart of patient care. In the UK, clinical radiologists work within the framework of the NHS as a close-knit team with radiographers, and in collaboration with many other specialties.

A Brief History

It is useful to have a background knowledge of the history of radiology as a specialty because interviewers will expect a basic level of understanding. As a relatively young specialty which has grown up alongside rapid advances in technology, it would not be unusual to be interviewed by radiologists who have experienced large changes in practice during their own careers. The following are some of the more important landmarks:

1895 - Wilhelm Roentgen discovers X-rays

1897 - The Roentgen Society is founded

1934 - The British Association of Radiologists (BAR) is founded

1962 - Kuhl introduces emission reconstruction tomography (later to become known as PET and SPECT)

1967 - The first clinical use of MRI takes place

1972 - Sir Godfrey Hounsfield supervises installation of the first prototype CT scanner at Atkinson Morley hospital

1975 - The Faculty of Radiologists becomes the Royal College of Radiologists

2010 - Interventional radiology is recognised as a radiology subspecialty

The College

The Royal College of Radiologists (RCR) governs the training and practice of radiology in the UK. Although it is a relatively young Royal College, it can trace its roots back to the Roentgen Society founded in 1897. It has been based at 63 Lincoln's Inn Fields in London since July 2013. Membership categories are as follows:

Category	Description
Associate	Those undertaking specialist training in clinical oncology or clinical radiology in the UK who have not yet passed the First FRCR Examination.

Junior	Those undertaking specialist training in clinical oncology or clinical radiology in the UK who have not yet passed the Final FRCR Examination.
Fellow	Those who have passed the Final FRCR Examination.

At interview you will be expected to know the main roles of the RCR which relate to training and quality assurance. These are namely:

- Setting the curriculum
- Examinations
- Issuing guidelines
- Representing radiologists in discussing national issues with the Department of Health

Current state of affairs

These days very few patients will leave hospital without undergoing some form of medical imaging, something which has placed the radiologist at the centre of the patient pathway. The demand for more radiologists has resulted in a growing number of opportunities for those who choose to train in the specialty, but has resulted in unique pressures upon the departments that provide imaging.

The RCR Annual Census is an important document to study during your interview preparation because it provides a summary of the radiology workforce in the UK and highlights important topics of debate. Key points include:

- There are an insufficient number of radiologists in the UK
- Between 2012-15, the number of CT and MRI scans increased by 26% and 29% respectively
- In 2015, 99% of UK radiology departments were unable to meet their reporting requirements, and 75% of departments outsourced some of their reporting work to private companies
- Since 2014, there has been a 51% increase in the annual radiology spend on outsourcing

Essentially, there is a mismatch between supply and demand in radiology. The exponential increase in the demand for medical imaging has not been matched by an increase in radiology training numbers. In order to increase workflow and maintain cost efficiency, radiology departments have employed a number of solutions. These are frequently referred to at interview, and we have listed some of the most important as 'hot topics'.

Hot topics

Outsourcing

Outsourcing is the external reporting of images by private companies. As NHS trusts struggle to keep up with the current volume of work, more imaging investigations are being reported by outside contractors to help meet demand and clear backlogs. Teleradiology refers to the method by which radiological images are transmitted between different locations and has been largely facilitated by the adoption of digital imaging, the internet and PACS. Outsourcing and teleradiology are favourite topics at interview, partly because radiologists differ widely on how they affect their specialty. You should be able to provide a balanced opinion on the subject and show understanding of the advantages and disadvantages.

The key document to read on this subject prior to interview is the RCR Teleradiology position statement (2015). The key message is summarised by the former RCR President Giles Maskell:

"The reporting of patients' images by a local radiologist who can speak directly to other clinicians is the best for patients. Remote reporting or teleradiology can provide a useful alternative when local services are over-stretched. However, patients deserve the reassurance that quality and safety are always the first priority, whoever reports their images. All radiologists who issue reports on UK patients should be subject to revalidation or an equivalent process regardless of where they are based."

Advantages of outsourcing include:
- Out-of-hours and emergency scans can be reported in a timely fashion in hospitals without a full on-call rota
- On-call reporting volumes can be reduced, allowing radiologists to provide a full in-hours service
- Specific investigations (e.g. plain films) can be outsourced, allowing in-house radiologists to concentrate on their own areas of expertise

Disadvantages include:
- Lack of training opportunities for in-house registrars if emergency scans are outsourced
- Outside radiologists may not have access to other clinical information (previous imaging, laboratory investigations), reducing the usefulness of their reports
- Outsourced reports are often reviewed in the morning or prior to MDTMs, leading to the phenomenon of 'double-reporting'
- Specialist work may be poorly reported

Essentially, the key is to provide a balanced view and to show that you have thought about the topic and discussed it with practicing radiologists. Should you lean towards one side of the fence, is important to be able to defend your opinion with reasoned arguments. However, your interviewer may have their own strong views on the matter, and so it may be wise to avoid controversy by giving an answer which is roughly in line with the RCR positon statement.

Skills mix

Skills mix refers to the reporting of images by non-radiologists. It often concerns advanced and consultant level radiographers training to report radiological investigations. Again, this has become more commonplace as radiology departments struggle to keep up with demand. Areas where it is most frequently seen are in x-ray reporting, breast screening and ultrasound. This is an important topic at interview because it is relevant to the future of the specialty as well as being reasonably contentious.

A key document covering this subject was released in 2012 by the RCR in conjunction with the Society and College of Radiographers (SoCR) entitled 'Team working in clinical imaging'. Essentially, it states that advanced practitioner or consultant radiographers - with appropriate training - should be allowed to report so long as it is subject to good governance and meets best practice standards. Again, the key here is to provide a balanced answer and to relate your views to what you have seen in practice. If it is something you have not experienced, shadowing a reporting radiographer in your hospital may give you a better idea. Just as with outsourcing, there are advantages and disadvantages of utilising skills mix.

Advantages include:
- Radiologist workload is reduced, especially in high-volume areas such as A&E x-ray reporting
- It is more cost-effective for radiology departments to employ radiographers to report rather than outsource
- Radiographers gain additional responsibility and may value the opportunity for extra career-progression

Disadvantages include:
- Difficult cases and ones outside the scope of the reporting radiographer will still need review by a radiologist
- Radiologists may still be accountable for work carried out by their radiographer colleagues
- Radiographer reporting may impact on training opportunities for radiology registrars

Turf wars

Turf wars refers to imaging procedures being carried out by other hospital specialties, and is often perceived as a threat to the field of radiology. For this reason, it is a subject which frequently comes up at interview. You should be able to list one or two examples of turf wars occurring between radiology and other specialties within the NHS, and how it may affect radiology services going forward. Try to be realistic but remain positive - there is more than likely plenty of work to keep radiologists busy for years to come.

In general, radiologists believe that they are the hospital specialty who should be reporting imaging studies and performing imaging guided procedures. After all, radiologists have expertise across all modalities, have knowledge of radiation and MR safety, and have training in spotting abnormalities outside of the primary field of interest. In the UK, and indeed outside, coronary angiography has long been performed by cardiologists. More recently, other areas of imaging including vascular intervention, emergency department ultrasound and cardiac MRI are being carried out largely by non-radiologists. Although this may worry a proportion of radiologists, advances in imaging technology mean that there are always new techniques to learn. Moreover, competition with other specialties can be seen as an incentive for radiologists to provide safer and more cost-effective services. Again, there are positives and negatives of other specialties undertaking the roles of radiologists:

Advantages include:
- Radiologist workload is reduced
- Other specialties may be in a better position to correlate imaging findings with clinical findings
- Other specialties may have more experience in certain areas (e.g. cardiologists in coronary angiography)

Disadvantages include:
- Radiologists risk losing interesting work
- Other specialties may miss pathology outside their fields of interest
- Other specialties have no formal training in physics or imaging safety

1.2 Radiology training

Radiology training in the UK is a 'run-through' training programme with a nationally coordinated recruitment process. It is a 5-year structured programme, although those wishing to subspecialise in interventional radiology must complete an additional 6th year of training.

Competition ratios

	2013	2014	2015	2016	2017
Applicants	754	794	917	963	937
Posts	210	229	244	249	262
Ratio	3.59	3.47	3.76	3.87	3.58

As the figures show, radiology is a competitive specialty and has a fairly stable competition ratio of just under four applicants per post. It is important to remember that these are national competition ratios and the most popular regions will themselves have higher competition ratios. We would advise not paying too much attention to the competition ratios and focus on how well you can score individually at interview.

Training programmes

There are 20 Local Education and Training Boards (LETBs)/Deaneries in the United Kingdom which you can apply to for training. Some of these are divided into two or more training schemes.

LETB/Deanery	Training Scheme(s)
East Midlands	Leicester; Nottingham
East of England	Cambridge, Essex & Bedfordshire; Norwich
KSS	Kent, Surrey & Sussex
London (North West)	Imperial; Chelsea & Westminster; Northwick Park
London (North Central & East)	Royal Free; Barts & the Royal London; University College Hospital
London (South)	Guy's and St Thomas'; King's College; St George's
North East	Newcastle upon Tyne; Teeside
North West	Manchester; Mersey
Northern Ireland MDTA	Northern Ireland
Scotland (East)	East Scotland (Dundee)
Scotland (North)	North Scotland (Aberdeen)

The Basics: 1.2 Radiology Training

Scotland (South East)	South East Scotland (Edinburgh)
Scotland (West)	West Scotland (Glasgow)
South West (Severn)	Bristol
South West (Peninsula)	Plymouth & Peninsula
Thames Valley	Oxford
Wales	South Wales; North Wales
Wessex	Portsmouth; Southampton
West Midlands	North Staffordshire, West Midlands (Birmingham)
Yorkshire and the Humber	Leeds/Bradford; Hull & East Yorkshire; Sheffield

Format of training

The path of standard training for a Certificate of Completion of Training (CCT) in clinical radiology is as follows (Clinical Radiology Curriculum, 2016):

- Primary Medical Qualification
- Foundation Years Training (FY1 and FY2) or equivalent with or without additional experience in other programmes (medicine, surgery etc.)
- Core Radiology Training (ST1-3) over a period of three years
- Advanced (special interest) Radiology Training (ST4-5) over a period of two years

Those applying to radiology training from Locum Appointment for Training (LAT) posts or Fixed Term Training Posts must have their original post approved by the GMC for it to count towards their training. Approval to count previous LAT training must be agreed by the College prior to starting a radiology training programme.

Although training structure differs between schemes, ST1-3 usually includes introductory blocks in major modalities such as CT and ultrasound as well as an introduction to the core sub-specialities including paediatrics, breast and neuroradiology. The final two years of training give the trainee an opportunity to focus on a specific area of interest. This structure is reflected in the RCR curriculum, which recognises core, level 1 and level 2 competencies. During the first three years of training, trainees are expected to achieve core competence (essentially what is expected of any radiologist performing acute/on-call imaging). During the last two years of training, trainees may go on to achieve level 1 or level 2 competencies in specific subject areas. By the end of training, a radiologist may hold level 1 in at least two areas (specialist interests), or level 2 in one area (as an expert in their field).

Delivery of training

Broadly speaking, the delivery of radiology training takes two formats: apprenticeship-style training and academy training. Most training schemes operate the more traditional apprenticeship-style in which the trainee is based within the department from day one. This gives the trainee early exposure to on-call reporting as well as the opportunity to work closely with senior radiologists and other clinicians. In 2005, a new style of radiology training was incorporated with the launch of three radiology academies; in Plymouth, Norwich and Leeds. This format of training involves much of the early curriculum content being delivered within a classroom environment and via e-learning. An important part of this is the Radiology Integrated Training Initiative (R-ITI) which is an e-learning resource launched by the College to support training.

Both styles of training have their advantages and disadvantages and it is up to the applicant to decide which is best suited to them. It is worth considering that the academy style of training is currently mandated by the RCR and those interviewing you may practice in such a scheme. It would therefore be wise to have some knowledge of how the academies work and provide a balanced opinion on the positives and negatives of training in one.

Advantages of academy training include:
- Exposure to numerous 'cold' cases which are hand-picked to demonstrate specific pathologies
- Freedom to make mistakes at an early stage of training
- Training can be standardised across schemes and set to match the RCR curriculum

Disadvantages include:
- A lack of early exposure to time-pressured or 'hot' reporting
- Difficulty delivering hands-on training such as intervention or ultrasound (although simulators are becoming available)
- Less time spent working with senior colleagues and other members of the department e.g. radiographers

E-Portfolio

No matter which training scheme you are a part of, the RCR ePortfolio will form a major part of your day-to day life as a trainee. The ePortfolio provides an electronic record of your progress and development through training and is evidence of your competence in specific areas of the RCR curriculum. Throughout training you will be expected to complete a mandatory number of workplace based assessments (WpBAs) in order to progress. These are recorded electronically in your ePortfolio and will be assessed at various points throughout the year. In radiology, WpBAs are slightly different than what you may be used to. They consist of:

1. Mini Image Interpretation Exercise (mini-IPX) – minimum of six per year
2. Radiology Direct Observation of Procedural Skills (RAD-DOPS) – minimum of six per year
3. Audit assessment – minimum of one per year
4. Teaching observation – minimum of two per year

5. Multisource feedback (MSF) – minimum of one per year
6. MDT assessment – minimum of two per year (after ST3)

In addition to WpBAs, you will be expected to undertake appraisals at the beginning and end of each clinical attachment. If, for instance, you complete an 8-week CT block during your ST1 year, you will be expected to complete two separate appraisals with your clinical supervisor to document your progress through the attachment.

Your WpBAs and appraisals will form the core of your Annual Review of Progression of Competence (ARCP) which takes place around July of each training year. During the ARCP, your ePortfolio evidence will be assessed to ensure that you are meeting the RCR curriculum objectives and can progress to the next level of training.

Examinations

Radiology is an exam-heavy specialty. It is important that applicants are aware of the added demands of training in such a specialty and have an up-to-date knowledge of the exam structure. The FRCR membership exam currently consists of two parts: the First FRCR Examination and the Final FRCR Examination.

First FRCR Examination

The First FRCR Examination will be your first major exam hurdle to navigate as a ST1. It ensures that you have a grounding in the physics that underpin modern diagnostic imaging and a good knowledge of the anatomy required to interpret radiological studies. It therefore comprises two modules: anatomy and physics. The anatomy image viewing module is delivered on individual workstations and physics is examined by a multiple choice question (MCQ) paper. Both modules are held on separate days, and you will be expected to attend the first sitting during March of your ST1 year. Both modules must be passed in order to progress to the Final FRCR. In the past, trainees were allowed unlimited attempts at the exam, however from 2015 it has been limited to six. Interviewers will expect you to pass well before your sixth attempt, and may ask you how you plan to prepare! In reality, most training schemes offer lectures and tutorials to help you to prepare, although awareness of the R-ITI e-learning modules will show an impressive amount of background knowledge. There are also a growing number of revision courses available, but from our experience there is simply no substitute for hard work!

Final FRCR Examination

The Final FRCR Examination comprises two parts: Part A and Part B.

Part A: This consists of two papers to be taken on the same day during your ST3 year. Questions are in single best answer (SBA) format and cover all aspects of clinical radiology. The single exam replaces the previous modular format which involved trainees sitting six separate papers. You will be expected to be aware of this change which was first announced by the RCR in 2015. Its purpose was to help trainees concentrate on other aspects of training rather than revise constantly for three or four years. Trainees are likely to have differing views on the change and so it may be useful to ask around in your local department.

Part B: This consists of a reporting session, a rapid reporting session and an oral examination. All components are examined via an image viewing session held in London twice a year. Candidates are required to have completed the Part A examination as well as have completed three years of training to be eligible.

1.3 The ST1 application overview

Mid-November – Early December	Application window via ORIEL
Mid-December	Specialty recruitment assessment (SRA) invitations
Mid-January	SRA window
Late January	SRA results and invitations to interview
Late February	Interview window
Early March	Initial offers

The Specialty Recruitment Assessment (SRA)

In 2016, recruitment into clinical radiology training changed with the introduction of the SRA. This brought radiology into line with several other specialty recruitment processes including ophthalmology and psychiatry. The SRA is a mandatory computer-based assessment which is used to shortlist candidates for interview. Further details are included in Chapter 2 of this book.

The ORIEL website recruitment portal

Recruitment into clinical radiology training is a nationally coordinated process. All applications must be submitted via the ORIEL recruitment website (www.oriel.nhs.uk). It is worth registering with ORIEL prior to the application window opening to familiarise yourself with the website. The system allows candidates to manage their application through a single portal and incorporates the following:

• An initial registration process meaning applicants only need one log-in for the entire recruitment year. Some parts of the completed registration will get transferred across to the application to avoid repeating information.

The Basics: 1.3 The ST1 Application Overview

- After registering, each applicant will have their own profile. It is through this that the applicant will complete the Clinical Radiology ST1 application form and be informed about developments with their application (invitations to the SRA and interview, programme offers etc.)
- Booking of the SRA and interview is managed through the portal
- All available vacancies for specialty training are listed on the website

The application

Applicants will make a single application via the ORIEL recruitment website during the job application window. You will be required to complete your personal details, employment history and medical qualifications. You must also declare any criminal convictions. You are required to provide referees; these should ideally be your most recent supervisors. It doesn't matter which speciality they work in, they will only be required complete the reference proforma if and when you are appointed an ST1 post.
It is important to be aware of the specific wording of the eligibility requirements and make sure you have copies of the required documents that will be checked on the day of the interview.

The initial longlisting of applications is conducted by London Recruitment. Eligibility is assessed against criteria on the clinical radiology person specification. Provided that you meet the required criteria, applicants will receive an email via the portal asking them to book a venue for the SRA which takes place in mid-January across a choice of times and venues. It is worth booking as soon as possible to ensure these are convenient for you.

Clinical radiology person specification

While the format and location of how applicants are selected into clinical radiology training have changed over the last few years, the underlying characteristics and desirable criteria for selection have not. The person specification outlines the requirements necessary for entry in clinical radiology training. The person specification is divided into two parts: entry criteria and selection criteria.

The entry criteria lists what is required to be eligible to apply for clinical radiology and this includes possessing a medical degree, having (or being expected to have) obtained your foundation training competencies, being in good health and being able to speak fluent English.

The selection criteria is the more important section as it is against this that applicants will be scored during interview. The selection criteria lists both 'essential' and 'desirable' criteria in certain domains together with the stage of the selection process these will be assessed and what evidence is required to score points. There are seven key domains against which applicants will be scored and it is important to be aware of these together with the 'desirable' criteria for each to know how to score maximum points during the selection process and what evidence may be required.

- Qualifications
- Clinical Experience
- Clinical Skills
- Academic Skills
- Personal Skills
- Probity
- Commitment to Speciality – Learning and Personal Development

Application structure

After registering through ORIEL candidates will be able to add information to the application system when it opens in Mid-November each year. The ORIEL application consists of 11 sections for clinical radiology. Each section is marked against the person specification and it is very important you compare your answers to this. Remember to fill in the application with care and do not leave it until the last minute. Every year there are examples of candidates who failed to make it through the longlisting stage because of this! The 11 sections are as follows:

1. Personal
2. Eligibility
3. Fitness
4. References
5. Competencies
6. Employment
7. Evidence
8. Supporting
9. Preferences
10. Equality
11. Declaration

It is worth noting that preferencing of individual training schemes is made available via ORIEL at a later stage of the application process prior to booking the interview. It is recommended that you only preference training schemes that you are willing to train and work in for the duration of your training.

1.4 The ST1 Interview Overview

There is no single part of the recruitment process that attracts more attention from applicants than the interview. However, despite the inevitable nerves which accompany it, this is your chance to show off and prove that you are the right candidate for the job. Invitations for interview are circulated in late-January based on SRA score, and interviews are held in London in late-February. Essentially, the key to interview success is thorough preparation, which ideally should begin long before your invitation to interview.

Structure

The interview structure has changed multiple times in recent years, adopting three different formats in as many years. In 2017, the interview consisted of three stations each lasting 10 minutes. Each station is assessed by two consultant interviewers, although there may also be a lay-person present to ensure that interviews are conducted in a fair manner.

In 2017, stations for the ST1 Clinical Radiology interview were:

- Preparation station (10 mins)
- Portfolio station (10 mins)
- Commitment to specialty station (10 mins)

Preparation station

At the start of the preparation station candidates were given an A4 mark sheet and asked to self-mark their portfolios. Five sections were included: clinical radiology experience, audits, teaching, exams and research. Candidates were asked to score themselves from 0 to 2 in each section based on their perceived level of achievement. The example scoring system given below is based on candidate feedback from the 2017 recruitment cycle and we feel is representative of what may come up in future years.

1. Clinical radiology experience

Clinical radiology experience	Score
1 or 2 full taster weeks/commitment to specialty beyond mandatory curriculum (>3 days)	2
Less than a full 1 week taster	1
No taster	0

2. Audit

Clinical audit	Score

A radiology audit/audit which made a difference or changed guidelines	2
Completed an audit which did not affect practice	1
No audit/poor quality audit	0

3. Teaching

Teaching	Score
Organised a teaching programme/completed a teaching diploma	2
Organised local teaching	1
Little/no teaching experience	0

4. Exams

Examinations	Score
Full MRCS/MRCP or equivalent within 4 years of graduation	2
Full MRCS/MRCP or equivalent after 4 years of graduation	1
No postgraduate exams	0

5. Research

Research	Score
Publication in more than one peer-reviewed journal/1st in intercalated BSc	2
Publication in one peer-reviewed journal/2:1 in intercalated BSc	1
No publication/additional degrees	0

Portfolio station

At the portfolio station two interviewers will ask you questions about different parts of your portfolio. There are no 'set' questions, rather questions are asked based on the scores you awarded to yourself during the preparation station. Questions will typically follow the five sections included on the A4 mark sheet: clinical radiology experience, audits, teaching, exams and research. It cannot be stressed enough just how important it is to be familiar with the person specification and please do refer to it when preparing answers for likely questions.

As scoring is done by comparison against the person specification, common questions can be prepared ahead of time. Given that interviewers will ask to see items of evidence contained within your portfolio, it is important that this is well-presented, key documents are easy to find and that you know the content well. In this chapter we will help you prepare your CV and portfolio to score maximum points at this station.

> **5 common portfolio station questions**
>
> These are some of the questions asked in the 2017 portfolio station. Chapter 3 of this book covers the portfolio station and features answers to these questions.
>
> 1. Take us through your CV
> 2. Tell us about an audit you have undertaken
> 3. Tell us about your teaching experience
> 4. Tell us about any postgraduate examinations you have completed
> 5. Tell us about any research you have been involved in

Commitment to specialty station

At the commitment to specialty station you will be asked about your experience of radiology and how your training so far has prepared you for a career in radiology. Candidates have remarked that this was the most open part of the interview, and interviewers will expect you to demonstrate an understanding of the specialty as a whole. You may be asked about the structure of radiology training including examinations and the ePortfolio. You will be expected to have some knowledge of the current issues facing radiology including outsourcing, skills mix and turf wars. It is important to relate all your answers back to your clinical radiology experience and what you have learned from radiology trainees and consultants. For instance, anyone can read about the FRCR exams online, but few will have taken the time to talk with radiology trainees about how they affect their training.

> **5 common commitment to specialty questions**
>
> These are some of the questions asked in the 2017 commitment to specialty station. Chapter 4 of this book covers the commitment to specialty station and features answers to these questions.
>
> 1. What is the role of the consultant radiologist?
> 2. What are the greatest challenges facing radiology?
> 3. What can you bring to radiology?
> 4. Tell us about radiology training
> 5. What do you think of skills mix?

Past interview stations

In past interviews, knowledge and skills and ethical scenarios stations have been included. It has historically been difficult to predict which stations will come up, and we recommend candidates be well prepared for any of these to be included again, particularly those included in the 2016 interview. To help with your interview preparation we have included a 2016 interview chapter which includes example questions from the previous recruitment year.

Knowledge and skills

In 2016, candidates were asked to critique a radiology report which they had been asked to read during the preparation station. Marks were awarded based on the candidates' critical analysis skills and understanding of what makes a good radiology report. See Chapter 5 for a more detailed explanation of this station. Prior to 2016, candidates were instead asked to read an audit summary which they were subsequently asked questions on.

Before 2016, candidates were asked to interpret images and prioritise imaging requests. Whilst these are important skills to develop as a radiologist, it is perhaps less likely that they will be included in future interviews as you are not expected to have any radiology-specific skills prior to starting training.

Ethical scenarios

Prior to 2017, an ethical scenarios station was included in the interview. This is likely to have been removed due to the introduction of the SRA, which tests ethical abilities. Even so, it is important to have a grasp of the ethical issues within radiology which include specific areas such as radiation protection and dealing with serious unexpected findings. These topics may appear in the commitment to specialty station to test your overall understanding of life in the radiology department. More generic topics such as professional behaviour, consent and dealing with difficult colleagues have also been tested. We have included a number of ethical scenarios along with model answers in Chapter 5.

1.5 The Radiological CV

There is no one correct way of ordering your CV and portfolio and ultimately you should structure it in a way that you are comfortable with so you can concisely sell your achievements during the portfolio station. What is certain however is that with there being just three stations in last year's interview, the portfolio station is now more important than ever and we present a suggested layout below to help maximise your marks from this station.

It is recommended that you use the same headings for your CV and portfolio. The CV should be a short summary of your achievements; not much more than a list of what you have done. This will help tick off the binary marks like qualifications and postgraduate examinations, but also act as a guide for finding further evidence in your portfolio when considering topics like audit, teaching and research which need more scrutiny for how many marks to award you. We will therefore consider the CV and portfolio together below.

Layout

The radiology application process is designed to assess you against the predefined person specification, so use this when thinking about how to lay out your portfolio. The following structure for your CV and portfolio encompasses the domains of the person specification to make it easy for your assessor to see that you are an excellent candidate for radiology.

Personal Details

Career Aspiration

1) **Qualification**
2) **Career History**
3) **Publications**
4) **Presentations**
5) **Awards & Prizes**
6) **Clinical Audit**
7) **Research Experience**
8) **Teaching**
9) **Management and Leadership**
10) **Development Courses & Conferences**
11) **Membership of Professional Organisations**
12) **Other Skills & Qualifications**
13) **Personal Interests**
14) **References**

Of course this is just a suggestion and if you are particularly strong in one area, for example if you have excellent teaching experience or have done a teaching qualification, it is probably worth prioritising this over audit or research.

Subheadings

Where possible, using neat subheadings under the main sections, will help make your CV even clearer and will make the interviewer think you are a well-organised, thorough candidate which are some of the characteristics on the person specification. For example, you could break the teaching section down

The Basics: 1.5 The Radiological CV

into 'national', 'local' and 'teaching courses/qualifications'.

Chronology

It is conventional on your CV to include the latest achievements at the top of the list. For example, in the presentations section, put your latest presentation at the top and any older ones beneath.

Content

Once you are happy with the structure of your CV and portfolio, you need to decide what to put in them. The nature of the radiology interview means you have both the CV and the portfolio at your disposal. You should therefore use both of these to maximise your performance at the interview. In our minds this means that the CV should act as a list of your entire achievements and help guide you and the interviewer to the correct area of your portfolio for more of an in-depth discussion about your achievements.

For example, if you included detailed descriptions about every aspect of each research project, audit, teaching episode and publication in your CV, it would be very long and potentially difficult to read. Simply listing your achievements in the CV with neat, standardised summaries of them in the relevant section of the portfolio is sensible and should lead to impressive, but clear and concise answers at interview when you are showing off what you have done. An example of an audit summary that you could include in your portfolio is shown below and similar summaries could be produced for research, teaching and management roles.

Title: Transabdominal ultrasound (US) scans in right upper quadrant (RUQ) abdominal pain: are we reporting these adequately?
Location: St Alexander's Hospital, London.
Background: Varying quality of US reports for RUQ pain locally.
My role in the audit: Identified the problem, led and designed audit, implemented change and re-audited.
Standard: Royal College of Radiologists guidelines on US reports.
Aim: 100% of reports to meet the defined standards.
Results: Just 50% of reports met the standards in their entirety.
Implementation: Local presentations of data. Consideration of structured reports – radiologists/radiographers reluctant, so listened to the feedback and used negotiating skills to place posters in reporting areas to ensure main standards commented on in reports.
Re-audit: 89% reports meet the defined standards.

Evidence

It can be tricky to know what evidence to include in your portfolio. This is increasingly important in the radiology interviews given the initial self-assessment of portfolios in the most recent interview. You need to prove what you claim!

For some things like postgraduate exams or qualifications, you can simply include the relevant certificate. For things like publications, put a printout of the paper in. For conference presentations, include a copy of the slides or the poster itself, together with proof of attendance at the conference. For audit, you should start with an audit summary like that listed above, but you should also include a copy of the slides from any presentation and evidence that you did it (like a registration with the local audit department or a certificate of completion). For research, you can include a succinct summary or abstract, together with any write-ups of your project. For teaching, include your teaching slides if you have them, any certificates and a summary of your feedback with some original examples.

With regards to evidence of feedback, this brings us on to another important area. Last year at the radiology interviews, a common question was about evidence of feedback about you. This could be in the form of 360-degree feedback from your colleagues at work, feedback from your supervisors or feedback from teaching or presentations you have done. It is certainly therefore worthwhile having summaries of feedback so you can talk about these and how you reflected on them and have changed for the better. It is also certainly worth including some negative feedback and some people were asked specifically for this. In terms of feedback about you professionally, perhaps this could be put in the 'Career History' section of the portfolio. This is also a good area to include evidence of reflection from your ePortfolio, which was another common question last year.

Radiology relevant

The ultimate goal of the radiology interview process is to pick out those candidates who genuinely want to do radiology and who will be well suited to the career. You should therefore focus your entire CV and portfolio towards radiology. Think carefully about whether including your GCSE results or maths Olympiad prize is important or whether they will just dilute your radiology focused achievements and make your CV/portfolio less concise. Of course, there are many non-radiological achievements that should be included which demonstrate important transferrable skills and show you are a well-rounded individual, but just be sensible when deciding what to include. Variety is key and the aim is to show that you are a well-rounded individual who is focused and determined to pursue radiology as a career.

Anything else to include?

Structuring the CV and portfolio in a manner similar to our suggestion should allow you to include all the important material. The only other thing we can think of that you may wish to include is a logbook of surgical, clinical or even radiological procedures. This could be included in the 'Career History' section or as a separate additional section in the portfolio that may not be needed in the CV. Radiology can be a very practical speciality, so showing evidence of practical skills is recommended.

Design

Formatting

It is recommended that you stick to a simple, consistent theme for both the CV and portfolio. Stick to a well-recognised, smart font like Arial or Times New Roman and be consistent with font sizes and formatting.

Index and dividers

Using an index based on the headings in your CV is a clear and sensible way to divide up your portfolio. Using labelled dividers will help you and the interviewer quickly navigate the portfolio.

Using page markers for carefully selected achievements can also be a helpful way of picking out achievements you are particularly proud of. Highlighting quotes from feedback that you have included will also help you talk about particular points and how you used this feedback to improve.

The portfolio itself

It is easy to be intimidated when on the day of the interview you are nervous and sit next to a candidate with an embossed, leather portfolio. In our opinion, it is not necessary to do this and a well-organised A4 ring binder with clear formatting throughout will be just as impressive. Ultimately it is about selling your achievements, with relevance to radiology, and you should be happy with a CV and portfolio that allows you to do this.

PRACTICAL TIPS FOR THE CV AND PORTFOLIO

- Prepare both your CV and portfolio a few weeks in advance of the interview– this helps ensure there are no last-minute printing issues and gives you ample time to….

- Practice quickly flicking through your portfolio with it upside down and you sat opposite an interviewer – from the authors' experiences this can be an unexpectedly tricky thing to do if you don't prepare for this!

- Practice sufficiently so that you know exactly where everything is and finding something is almost second nature in the interview

- Get colleagues, friends and family to read through your CV and portfolio for feedback and to ensure they do you justice

The Basics: 1.5 The Radiological CV

> **Helpful articles for preparing a medical CV can be found at:**
> http://careers.bmj.com/careers/advice/Preparing_the_perfect_medical_CV
> http://careers.bmj.com/careers/advice/Preparing_your_medical_CV
> https://www.bma.org.uk/advice/career/applying-for-a-job/medical-cv

Example CV for a Radiology Interview

Curriculum Vitae: John Smith

Address: 10 Colverville Road, London, SW10 5PN	Date of birth: 23/04/91
Telephone: 12345689 Email: johnsmith@johnsmith.ac.uk	GMC: 1234567

Foundation Year 2 Doctor

Career Aspiration

Develop a successful career in the field of radiology through combining clinical work with academia.

1.) Qualifications
Postgraduate
Intercollegiate MRCS Part A	81.2%, April 2016
Advanced Trauma and Life Support	The Royal Hospital, Canterbury, February 2016
Advanced Life Support	The Royal Hospital, Canterbury, September 2015

Undergraduate
Medicine (MBChB) 2009-2015:	University of Canterbury - Graduated with distinction
Physiological Sciences (BSc) 2011-2012:	University of Canterbury - Upper second class honours

2.) Career History
Foundation Programme
Foundation Year 2 Doctor - St Alexander's Hospital, London.
Educational Supervisor: Dr Tim Watson	August 2016-August 2017
Post 1) Cardiology - Dr Helen Robertson	
Post 2) Emergency Medicine - Dr Niall Dobson	
Post 3) Vascular Surgery - Mr Tony Thompson	August 2015-August 2016

Foundation Year 1 Doctor - The Royal Hospital, Canterbury.
Educational Supervisor: Dr Manoj Sharma
Post 1) Upper GI Surgery - Mr Ishaan Malhi
Post 2) Medicine for the Elderly - Dr Sheila Robson
Post 3) Diabetes and Endocrinology - Dr Stephanie Rogers

Radiology experience
Taster week - St Alexander's Hospital, London.
Supervisor: Dr John Jones
Taster days - The Royal Hospital, Canterbury.
Supervisor: Dr Helena Robertson

3.) Publications
Peer-reviewed Journals
Wardle AW, **Smith J**, Johnson MD. MRI findings of sickle cell disease. British Journal of Musculoskeletal Radiology 2016;52(3): 310-18.

Smith J, Arter J, Goff M. Shared medical appointments for vascular surgery follow-up. Journal of Vascular Medicine 2014;23(7): 100-20.

Published Abstracts
Smith J, Jones R, Wijesekera R. Radiological investigation of renal/ureteric lithiasis with CTKUB. British Journal of Imaging 2016;75(Supplement 1): S13-14.

Smith J, Suliman R, Effron J, Sykes S. The diagnostic utility of "out of hours" computed tomography of the head at a District General Hospital. French Journal of Surgery 2015;131(S1): 126-127.

4.) Presentations
Oral - International & National
Smith J, Jones R, Wijesekera R. Radiological investigation of renal/ureteric lithiasis with CTKUB. 51st British Imaging Symposium, 16-17th April 2016, London, UK.

Oral - Local
Smith J - Adrenal Incidentalomas. Endocrinology Department Teaching 5th July 2016, The Royal Hospital, Canterbury, UK.
Smith J, Patel R. Diabetes Integrated Care Canterbury Launch Event. 24th May 2016, Welling Hall, Canterbury, UK.

Poster - International & National
Smith J, Timmins L, Ramsay R, Johnson J. Safety and diagnostic accuracy of transrectal prostate biopsy in a District General Hospital setting. 13th British Symposium on Urogenital Radiology. 15th-16th July 2016, Leeds, UK.
Smith J, Suliman R, Effron J, Sykes S. The diagnostic utility of "out of hours" CT of the head at a District General Hospital. The Annual French Radiology Meeting, 15th-18th September 2016, Paris, France

The Basics: 1.5 The Radiological CV

5.) Awards & Prizes
Postgraduate
Runner-up of the Foundation Doctor Essay Award - The Foundation Programme
Undergraduate
2013 Undergraduate Elective 1st Prize - The Clinical Society of Canterbury, The Clinical Society President's Meeting
Grants & Bursaries
Undergraduate Elective Bursary - The Clinical Society of Canterbury
Elective Bursary - University of Canterbury

6.) Clinical Audit
Transabdominal ultrasound (US) scans in right upper quadrant (RUQ) abdominal pain: are we reporting these adequately? -St Alexander's Hospital, London
Radiological Investigation of Renal Colic with CTKUB - The Royal Hospital, Canterbury
The diagnostic utility of "out of hours" computed tomography of the head - The Royal Hospital, Canterbury

7.) Research Experience
Shared medical appointments for vascular surgery follow-up - Student Selected Component (SSC) Project, The Royal Hospital, Canterbury. Supervisor: Mr Martin Goff. Funding: None.
The role of SAG12 in fertility - BSc Dissertation Project, Microvascular research laboratories, University of Canterbury. Supervisor: Professor Hannah Elias. Funding: British Fertility Foundation (PG/08/033/26282, BS/06/5) & Wellcome Trust (45029) grants.

8.) Teaching
Teaching Experience - National
Fit 4 Finals Revision Courses Programme Leader - National Teaching, lecture based. Organised 2 courses and delivered radiology for finals lectures.

Teaching Experience - Local
Chest X-rays – The Royal Hospital, Canterbury. Interactive lecture to 3rd & 4th year medical students.
University of Canterbury Year 3 Medical Student Tutor – The Royal Hospital. Delivered abdominal radiograph lecture, bedside teaching & tutorials.
Mock Data Objective Structure Clinical Examination Organiser - University of Canterbury. Organised mock exam for medical students.
Spanish GCSE Tutor - Canterbury. Tutored A level student Spanish.

Teaching Courses
Introduction to Problem Based Learning in the Faculty of Medicine - Educational Development Unit (EDU), University of Canterbury
Introduction to Feedback and Formative Assessment - EDU, University of Canterbury

9.) Management & Leadership

Fit 4 Finals Revision Courses Programme Leader - Fit 4 Finals
British Medical Association Local Negotiating Committee Junior Doctor representative - The Royal Hospital, Canterbury
University of Canterbury Medical Society Committee Member - University
Bar Representative - University of Canterbury

10.) Development Courses & Conferences
Radiology
Introduction to Radiology - Stafford Radiology Academy, Stafford
Interventional Radiology Trainee Day – The Interventional Radiologists of Great Britain and Ireland (IRGBI), Liverpool
Top Tips for ED Radiology - Radiology Courses, London
Other
Management and Leadership Skills for Foundation Doctors - London Deaner

11.) Membership of Professional Organisations
- British Imaging Society Foundation Member
- IRGBI Foundation Member
- Trainee Radiologists Society
- British Medical Association

12.) Other Skills & Qualifications
- Proficient user of Microsoft Office and Graphpad Prism statistical software
- Post-graduate Spanish for medical studies (score 76%) – a year 2 SSC (2010/11)

13.) Personal Interests
- Sport - 1st XV school rugby team & Medical School team. I follow football, rugby & cricket
- Travelling, cinema, food, reading & diving

14.) References
- Dr Tim Watson, Consultant Gastroenterologist, Department of Gastroenterology, St Alexander's Hospital, London. Telephone: 123456789, fax: 123456789.
Email: tim.watson@stalex.nhs.uk
- Mr Ishaan Malhi, Consultant General Surgeon, Department of General Surgery, The Royal Hospital, Canterbury. Telephone: 123456789, fax: 123456789.
Email: ishaan.malhi@rhc.nhs.uk
- Dr Manoj Sharma Consultant Cardiologist, Department of Cardiology, The Royal Hospital, Canterbury. Telephone: 123456789, fax: 123456789.
Email: manoj.sharma@rhs.nhs.uk

1.6 Interview Technique

Making an impression and scoring highly at the interview stations is as much about your overall interview technique as it is about the content of your answers. Coming across as confident and a 'good' candidate is a skill and can be improved with practise. Try to utilise the below interview techniques when practising your answers.

1.6.1 Interview Communication Skills

Interviews are not just about facts and it is important that you are aware of other factors that will contribute to your interview score and the overall impression that you leave the interviewers with.

Body language (Non-Verbal Communication Skills)

Body language is extremely important and plays a pivotal role in effective communication. It can be difficult to know how to sit, who to look at or what to do with your arms during an interview.

Sitting
A number of studies have identified the position of sitting slightly forward feet planted on the ground with hands crossed or fingers locked and forearms resting on your thighs as being the optimum position for interviews. This position makes you look calm and ready and is in between leaning over the table and slouching back in your chair. This position can be maintained for the majority of the interview and allows you to sit back slightly between questions or at the end of the interview.

Smile
Smiling has been shown to increase attractiveness by a factor of ten and will also convey confidence and personality to the interviewers. While you may be extremely nervous make sure you smile when you greet the panel and try to show enthusiasm when talking about why you want to be a radiologist and the things you have done.

Eye Contact
Ensure that you make eye contact with the interviewers from the start. If you find holding eye contact difficult practice focussing on peoples' eyebrows when you talk to them (the eye of the other person cannot discriminate whether you are looking at their eye or eyebrow due to proximity). When listening to questions concentrate on the interviewer asking the questions, nodding to show understanding. When giving your answers make sure you make eye contact with all the panel and not just the interviewer asking the question. At least one of the interviewers will be making notes or scoring you so do not be phased if they do not maintain eye contact.

The Basics: 1.6 Interview Technique

Hands
From the initial handshake to using hand gestures to enforce points your hands can help to demonstrate confidence and conviction if used correctly. Upon entering the room respond to handshakes if offered and look the interviewers in the eyes. Keep your hands on your knees or lap when listening to questions and raise them when making a firm point.

Appearance
For male applicants: smart shoes, smart suit, plain shirt and plain tie. For women a smart skirt or trousers and a shirt with or without a suit jacket will be fine.

Active Listening
When being asked questions sit attentively. Movements such as tilting your head or nodding in understanding demonstrate active listening and will make you appear more engaging to the interviewers.

Verbal Communication Skills

Once you have mastered body language it is time to analyse how you deliver your responses to the interviewers. An excellent answer delivered in a quiet, stuttering manner will score less than one given with gusto.

Vocal Clarity
Project your voice beyond the interviewers, sit upright and speak clearly. You will be nervous initially and may hear your voice waiver. This is entirely normal and you will settle in to things after you begin speaking.

Length of Response
Stopping yourself from talking when nervous can be extremely difficult, however, interviewers are likely to lose concentration after around 3 minutes of listening to you talk. Most structured points can be given within 2-3 minutes leaving time for further questions.

Speed
Some people talk quickly others talk slowly. Try to find a balance and don't be afraid to pause to consider the question before jumping into your answer.

Vocal Tonality
Changing your inflection and emphasising words prevents interviewers from getting bored. Think about how quickly you lose interest when speaking to someone talking about something in a monotonous, single tone voice and then think about someone who changes their tone and emphasises words. Less easy to fall asleep, right?

Enthusiasm
Following on from tonality and word emphasis make sure that you are enthusiastic when delivering your answers. Smiling and tonality make up a large portion of this and the rest is about overcoming nerves and remembering that you should be excited about radiology and the things that you have done.

The Basics: 1.6 Interview Technique

Positive Answers
When answering structured, portfolio questions be sure to turn everything into a positive even when asked about weaknesses or receiving criticism. Take a look at the list of action words at the end of this chapter for more examples of how to verbally demonstrate confidence.

✎ Vocal Tonality Practice

The sentence 'I want to be a radiologist' can be interpreted in a number of ways depending on the tonality of the delivery. For instance a person increasing their inflection towards the end of the sentence suggests a question: 'I want to be a radiologist?'. While delivery with a firm tone suggests more of a statement: 'I want to be a radiologist!'. More over emphasis of words can dramatically alter the sentence structure; 'I WANT to be a radiologist', 'I want to BE A RADIOLOGIST'.

TOP TIPS

➕ **Confidence:** Smile, make eye contact, project your voice and use positive language to convey confidence when answering questions.

➕ **Keep To The Point:** Keep your answers short and make sure you directly answer the question posed.

1.6.2 Interview Frameworks

Although you cannot predict and prepare for every question that might be asked at interview it is helpful to have a framework to answer specific portfolio-type questions. Roughly speaking questions asked at any type of interview can be categorised into motivational, situational, opinion and specific. Having a framework will help you to logically structure your answers for both basic and more challenging questions and help you think under pressure.

Different question types will require different frameworks. Question types fall into categories or domains based on what the interviewers are testing. Whichever framework you use you should be able to cut your answer down to 3-4 solid, personal experiences and reflect on each. Remember these frameworks are guides only and it is fine to use a different way to structure your answer or only use part of the framework. You can find examples of these frameworks in action in the portfolio chapter.

Motivational and Experiential: CAMP

E.g. Why radiology? Tell me About Your Work Experience

Clinical
Academic
Management
Personal

Problem-Solving Questions: SPIES

E.g. How would you deal with this problem?

Situation
Problem
Initiative
Escalate
Support

Situational and Skills Questions: STAR

E.g. How have you shown leadership? Have you been part of a team?

Situation
Task
Action
Result

The Basics: 1.6 Interview Technique

1.6.3 Interview Circuit Technique

It is important to remember that you will be rotating around an interview circuit with other candidates behind and ahead of you. Your starting station will be random and there is no 'good' or 'bad' first station. If you think an interview station has not gone as well as you had hoped don't dwell on it as you will be going directly into a new station afterwards. Below are some further tips specific for the OSCE-style of interview.

Don't Forget to...

Read The Question: Ensure you read or listen to each question and understand what the interviewers want from your answer.

Keep to Time: Make sure your answers are succinct and focussed. Time is limited as you will be moving stations and there will be little time to waffle on.

Remain Calm: If a station goes badly forget about it, don't panic and give the next station your best shot.

Be Confident: If you follow the advice in this book and practise the questions contained within you will be well-prepared. By the time the interviews come round there will be nothing more you can do and you should feel confident and focus on your interview technique.

Content of Answers

Regardless of the interview type, interviewers will want to know about your experience, your extracurricular activities, how you deal with pressure, how you resolve problems and whether you can demonstrate empathy.

Be Personal and Specific: Talking about generic things like 'I saw a patient having blood taken' or 'I have leadership skills' will not score you as many points as using personal experiences and reflecting on what you learned.

Structure Your Answers: Structuring your answers into 3-4 headlines will make it easy for interviewers to follow and prevent you from wasting time with waffle.

Common Questions: Write out example answers for common questions and then practise them. Try not to be too scripted rather work on your delivery and enthusiasm once you are happy with your content.

Use Your CV As A Guide: Interviewers may have missed key parts of your CV or portfolio. Make sure that you talk about all the best points that you have written down and do not assume that the interviewers have read it. Your CV should be structured to say why you want to do radiology, what work experience you have done and what you know about radiology training.

The Basics: 1.5 Interview Technique

Show Your Working: For decision-making questions be sure to talk through what you are thinking. There is often no right or wrong answer rather the interviewers want to see you logically discussing both sides of the argument or problem.

Be Positive and Sell, Sell, Sell: Interviewers want to hear how great you are and it is important that you are not bashful or reserved when telling them about your achievements and why they should choose you. Turn everything into a positive and don't undersell yourself.

Don't Give An Overview: Outlining how you are going to answer a question or explaining your framework is unnecessary and risky. One particularly awkward moment occurred when an interview candidate confidently stated there were three reasons he wanted to be a radiologist only for him to be unable to recall the third!

Answer The Question: This might seem silly but it is amazing how often candidates do not give a direct answer or go off-topic. Make sure you understand what has been asked and avoid giving a long-winded introduction.

Other Factors

The thought of the interview can be scary and there are some other variables that you will need to consider such as how you are going to get to the venue and what happens when you get there. You will be sent detailed information regarding the interview process and venue in good time. Below are some top tips for how to stay calm around the time of the interview itself.

The Night Before: You may have chosen to stay in the city before your interview or you may be travelling up on the day. Whatever you have chosen to do ensure that you have your clothes prepared, shoes shined and know where and when you need to be at the interview location. Ensure you have all the required documentation and identification required well ahead of time. Relax and get a good night's sleep the evening before, making sure you set your alarm to wake up in good time the next morning.

On the Day: Get up in good time and have a proper breakfast. Make sure you factor in traffic if you are driving to the interview location. Upon arriving at the venue you will need to register so that the organisers know that you have arrived. Occasionally your interview time slot may have been altered. If this is the case don't panic and go with the flow. There will be refreshments provided and you will be told where you can wait before the interview.
An interviewer or facilitator will usually call you in once they are ready. Upon entering greet the interviewers ensuring that you try to appear as confident as possible.

1.6.4 What The Interviewers Say

We asked a selection of experienced interviewers to give their opinions on what makes the difference between a good candidate and an excellent candidate. Here is what they had to say:

> "The biggest challenge of any interview candidate is answering the questions posed in a way that incorporates your best points in a concise format. Your interview station time is limited. This can be especially difficult when asked a very broad, open question such as 'Why should we choose you?'"

> "As an interviewer I can tell you that the best candidates are the ones who answer the questions posed in a logical and structured format and who have clearly thought about how they will answer the common questions."

> "Candidates who appear confident, with good body language and vocal intonation have often acquired this through previous interview or public speaking experiences. The more formal interview practice that you do the more relaxed you will be on the day of the real thing and this will translate into a more confident performance."

> "Ask any interviewer what separates the best and worst interview candidates and they are likely to respond with a single word 'waffle'. (Most) interviewers are human and will be interviewing candidates for the entire day of interviews. Think about the last time you spoke with someone, maybe a friend or relative, who told a long and boring story. It can be difficult to stay focused and retain information when candidates talk for longer than 3-4 minutes or repeat themselves. Preparing and practising questions with a set framework will help you to get across your best selling points in a concise format."

> "Some candidates struggle to sell themselves and feel awkward or boastful when asked why they would be a good doctor or why they should be chosen. The best way around this is to bring objectivity into the answer. For example, rather than saying 'I am a great leader' you may be more comfortable saying 'feedback from my supervisors and peers highlights my strong leadership skills'."

1.6.5 CV and Interview Action Words

One way to really sell yourself in both your application and interview is to make sure you choose appropriate action words that match the corresponding skills that are being assessed.

Below is a list of action words that you may wish to use when writing your application and CV and when answering interview questions to make your answers sound more positive and assertive.

Leadership Skills

Administered
Appointed
Approved
Assigned
Attained
Authorized
Chaired
Considered
Consolidated
Contracted
Controlled
Converted
Coordinated
Decided
Delegated
Developed
Directed
Eliminated
Emphasized
Enforced
Enhanced
Established
Executed
Generated
Handled
Headed
Hired
Hosted
Improved
Incorporated
Increased
Initiated
Inspected
Instituted
Led
Merged
Motivated
Originated
Overhauled
Oversaw
Planned
Presided
Prioritized
Produced
Recommended
Reorganized
Replaced
Restored
Reviewed
Scheduled
Streamlined
Strengthened
Supervised
Terminated

Communication Skills

Addressed
Advertised
Arbitrated
Arranged
Articulated
Authored
Clarified
Collaborated
Communicated
Composed
Condensed
Conferred
Consulted
Contacted
Conveyed
Convinced
Corresponded
Debated
Defined
Described
Developed
Directed
Discussed
Drafted
Edited
Elicited
Empathised
Enlisted
Explained
Expressed
Formulated
Furnished
Incorporated
Influenced
Interacted
Interpreted
Interviewed
Involved
Joined
Lectured
Listened
Mediated
Moderated
Negotiated
Observed
Outlined
Participated
Persuaded
Presented
Promoted
Proposed
Publicized
Reconciled
Recruited
Referred
Reinforced
Reported
Resolved
Responded
Solicited
Specified

Spoke
Suggested
Summarized
Synthesized
Translated

Research Skills

Analysed
Clarified
Collected
Compared
Conducted
Critiqued
Detected
Determined
Diagnosed
Evaluated
Examined
Experimented
Explored
Extracted
Formulated
Gathered
Identified
Inspected
Interpreted
Interviewed
Invented
Investigated
Located
Measured
Organized
Researched
Searched
Solved
Summarized
Surveyed
Systematized
Tested

Teaching Skills

Adapted
Advised
Clarified
Coached
Communicated
Conducted
Coordinated
Critiqued
Developed
Enabled
Encouraged
Evaluated
Explained
Facilitated
Focused
Guided
Individualized
Informed
Instilled
Instructed
Motivated
Persuaded
Set Goals
Simulated
Stimulated
Taught
Tested
Trained
Transmitted
Tutored

Helping Skills

Adapted
Advocated
Aided
Answered
Assessed
Assisted
Clarified
Coached
Collaborated
Contributed
Cooperated
Counselled
Demonstrated
Educated
Encouraged
Ensured
Expedited
Facilitated
Familiarize
Insured
Intervened
Motivated
Provided
Referred
Rehabilitated
Presented
Resolved
Simplified
Supplied
Supported
Volunteered

Organisational and Management Skills

Approved
Arranged
Catalogued
Categorized
Charted
Classified
Coded
Collected
Compiled
Corresponded
Distributed
Executed
Filed
Generated
Implemented
Incorporated
Inspected
Logged
Maintained
Monitored
Obtained
Operated
Ordered
Organized
Prepared
Processed
Provided
Purchased
Recorded
Registered
Reserved
Responded
Reviewed
Routed
Scheduled
Screened
Set Up
Submitted

2 SRA

2.1 Introduction to the SRA 42
2.2 Professional Dilemmas *(PD/SJT)* 43
2.3 Clinical Problem Solving *(CPS)* 50

2.1 Introduction To The SRA

The SRA stands for the Specialty Recruitment Assessment. It was introduced to the ST1 recruitment process in 2016, brining clinical radiology into line with other specialties including psychiatry and ophthalmology. The SRA is a mandatory computer-based assessment which is used primarily to shortlist candidates for interview. It consists of two parts: A Professional Dilemmas (PD/SJT) paper and a Clinical Problem Solving (CPS) paper. According to the RCR (2017):

"IIn line with a number of other specialties a Specialty Recruitment Assessment (SRA) test was incorporated into radiology recruitment in 2016. All applicants are required to sit the SRA at a test centre in the January of the recruitment year. Applicants are ranked according to their SRA score and invitations to interview are circulated on the basis of rank until all available 600 interview slots are filled. Full details of the test, including the available test venues in the UK and overseas, will be published on the ORIEL recruitment system when applications open."

How, when and where

All applicants meeting the eligibility criteria set out in the person specification will be required to sit the SRA. Invitations will be sent via the ORIEL website application portal in mid-December. Attendance is mandatory and the test can be taken within a set window - usually mid-January - at Pearson VUE Centres across the country. You will be given a choice of times and venues, and so it is important to respond early to ensure these are convenient for you.

Format

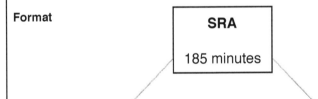

SRA

185 minutes

Professional Dilemmas (PD/SJT)

- Ranking
- Multiple choice

58 questions in 110 minutes

Clinical Problem Solving (CPS)

- Extended matching questions (EMQ)
- Multiple best answer (MBA)
- Single best answer (SBA)

97 questions in 75 minutes

2.2 Professional Dilemmas (PD/SJT)

Professional Dilemmas (PD/SJT)

This paper consists of 58 questions to be completed in 110 minutes. Questions are presented in Situational Judgement Test (SJT) format, similar to the style used in Foundation Programme recruitment. It is not a test of your knowledge, but of your behaviours and attitudes in the workplace with respect to interacting with colleagues and patients and managing your workload. Responses are expected at the level of a FY2 doctor. Three core domains are covered:

1. Professional integrity
2. Coping with pressure
3. Empathy and sensitivity

Your responses will be scored based on how close they are to the most appropriate response for each question (based on the responses of a group of experts). Provided that your answers are close to the most appropriate responses you will still be able to score highly. The minimum score for ranking responses completely out of order is eight marks, and so it is important to attempt to rank every response. Failure to rank responses will result in a score of zero for that question. Only 50 questions will count towards the final score, as eight questions are for piloting purposes only.

There are two specific question formats:

1. Rank five possible responses in order

Examples

I. You are coming to the end of your shift on the Medical Assessment Unit (MAU). Your FY2 colleague who you are due to hand over to informs the nursing staff he is running 30 minutes late. You are meeting a friend for dinner that evening and are keen not to leave work late.

Rank in order the following actions to this situation (1=Most appropriate; 5=Least appropriate).

A. Let your friend know that you will be 30 minutes late for dinner
B. Make a list of outstanding jobs, leave this on the nurse's station and leave at the end of your shift
C. Make a list of outstanding jobs and give to your colleague as soon as he arrives so that you can leave the hospital
D. Do a quick round of the ward, detail all outstanding issues relating to each patient in their notes and leave at the end of your shift
E. Make a list of outstanding jobs and give to your registrar to hand to your colleague when he arrives for his shift

Answer: ACEDB

Option A is the most desirable option because it ensures safe and effective handover. Staying 30 minutes late on a single occasion is acceptable given the circumstances, however should be escalated if it is a recurring event. Option C ensures that your colleague receives written handover, although it is preferable to stay for a few minutes to handover verbally as well. Option E is similar, yet involves your registrar remembering to give the job list to your colleague. Options D and B are the least desirable as it is unlikely your colleague will realise there are jobs to be done and patient care may suffer as a result. Option B puts patient information in a potentially public space and is therefore worse than option D.

II. You are the FY2 doctor on-call for surgery. You are asked to consent a patient for an emergency appendicectomy. You have read about the procedure but you have never seen one before.

Rank in order the following actions to this situation (1=Most appropriate; 5=Least appropriate).

A. Refuse and wait for somebody else to do it.
B. Complete the consent form with the patient and omit mentioning any complications you are not aware of.
C. Discuss the procedure with your registrar and ask her to observe you carrying out consent.
D. Ask your registrar for more information on the procedure.
E. Carry out consent with one of the other Foundation doctors and hope they can answer the patient's questions.

Answer: CDEBA

Option C allows the registrar to answer any questions the patient may have whilst enabling you to learn more about the consent process and is therefore the best option. Option D is beneficial for your learning although you may still not be able to answer all of the patient's questions. Option E shows that you have asked for help, albeit from another inexperienced member of the team who be no more knowledgeable than you. Option B shows that you have attempted to complete the task but you have not given the patient the information they need to know. Option A is the least desirable option because you have not attempted to deal with the issue which may cause a delay with the operation.

III. You are the orthopaedic FY2 about to begin the morning ward round. Your consultant arrives on the ward smelling strongly of alcohol and slurring his words slightly. You have heard from the nursing staff that he is going through a divorce.

Rank in order the following actions to this situation (1=Most appropriate; 5=Least appropriate).

A. Call the GMC to formally report the doctor
B. Ask your registrar to take your consultant away from the ward whilst you continue the ward round
C. Quietly take the consultant to one side and ask him to leave the ward before continuing the ward round with your registrar
D. Say nothing because he is probably going through a difficult time and things will get better
E. Tell the ward clerk what you think is going on

Answer: CBAED

Option C is the best option because it deals directly with the threat to patient safety should your consultant continue the ward round. Option B is taking responsibility away from you, which is not best practice, however your registrar is likely to be in a good position to deal with the situation. Option A is harsh but makes sure that the situation is dealt with, albeit not immediately. Option E is not a good option as the ward clerk is not best placed to deal with the issue and may result in further harm being done to your consultant's reputation. Option D is the worst option because it does not attempt to deal with the situation and compromises patient safety.

IV. During your GP rotation, you see a 62-year-old chauffeur to review his recently started antiepileptic medication. During your last consultation you told him he could no longer drive, however you saw him arrive today in his car. You are aware from other patients that he is continuing to work as a chauffeur.

Rank in order the following actions to this situation (1=Most appropriate; 5=Least appropriate).

A. Do nothing, as he might get upset and not return to the practice
B. Phone the DVLA immediately and report him
C. Inform him that because he has ignored your previous advice, you have no choice but to inform the DVLA
D. Continue the consultation and remind him at the end that he should not be driving and should contact the DVLA
E. Phone his wife and get her to ask him to stop

Answer: CBDEA

In this situation, you are left with no choice but to inform the DVLA as the patient poses a risk both to himself and to the public by continuing to drive. Option C is the most desirable option because you are keeping the patient informed of your actions. Option B is the next most desirable because you are still informing the DVLA, albeit without the patient's knowledge or consent. Option D would be a reasonable first step, however the scenario states that the patient has ignored past warnings and is likely to do so again. Option E shows that you are concerned, but breaks confidentiality and might damage the doctor-patient relationship further. Option A is the least desirable as you are ignoring the problem.

SRA: 2.2 Professional Dilemas

V. Towards the end of your GP rotation, a patient who you have been treating at the practice and have developed a good rapport with hands you a box containing a gold watch. She asks you to keep it as a token of her gratitude.

Rank in order the following actions to this situation (1=Most appropriate; 5=Least appropriate).

A. Thank the patient but tell her that you cannot possibly accept the gift
B. Tell the patient that it is inappropriate and hand it straight back
C. Keep the watch and don't make a record
D. Keep the watch but make a record on your electronic portfolio
E. Give the watch to the lead partner at the practice

Answer: ADEBC

The GMC state that you must not accept gifts that may affect or be seen to affect the way you prescribe for or treat patients. In the case of a gold watch, this is in excess of what would be expected as a token of appreciation. Option A is the most desirable option as you are maintaining the doctor-patient relationship whilst politely declining the gift. Option D is the next best option because the patient will not be offended and a record of the gift is available to maintain probity. The lead partner at the practice is good person to ask for advice, however giving them the watch does not guarantee they will do the right thing (Option E). Option B avoids the potential pitfalls of accepting a gift but may be unnecessarily damaging to the doctor-patient relationship as the gift is likely well-meaning. Option C is dishonest and shows a lack of probity.

2. Select the three most appropriate responses

Examples

I. You are a FY2 doctor working in orthopaedics. You have just given a teaching presentation to a group of final year medical students. Your consultant tells you that feedback from the medical students was poor.

Choose the **THREE most appropriate** *actions to take in this situation.*

A. Do more reading on the subject matter to prepare next time
B. Ask your consultant for more detailed feedback
C. Ask for feedback from your FY2 colleagues on your teaching skills
D. Arrange for further training on presentation skills
E. Ask a colleague to help you practice for your next teaching session
F. Opt out of future teaching sessions as it is not one of your strengths
G. Write a reflective entry on the situation in your Foundation portfolio
H. Ask your consultant to observe your next teaching session

Answers: B, D, H

Option B is an important first step because it will help you to understand which areas of your teaching are currently deficient. Your consultant will be in a good position to relay feedback from the medical students and can advise you on how to make improvements. Option D shows that you are proactive and keen to improve. Teaching skills are an important part of the job and you should always seek opportunities to learn. By asking your consultant to observe your next teaching session (Option H) you are actively seeking feedback from a knowledgeable source and could go on to include this is your electronic portfolio.

II. You review a patient on the orthopaedic ward who has recently undergone surgery for a fractured neck of femur. You write a prescription for strong painkillers, however the nursing staff challenge your decision and refuse to give the medication.

Choose the **THREE most appropriate** *actions to take in this situation.*

A. Review the patient again
B. Arrange to speak to the nurse later to discuss your working relationship
C. Ask a more senior nurse to give the medication
D. Ask a senior colleague for advice
E. Complete an incident form
F. Prescribe paracetamol instead
G. Tell the patient that the nurse has refused to give the medication
H. Discuss with the nurse why she disagrees with your prescription

Answer: A, D, H

Option A shows that patient safety is your main priority in this scenario. By reviewing the patient again, you are ensuring that there is nothing you have missed and that the patient still requires the medication. Option D is also a sensible option as there has been a disagreement regarding patient care and senior input may be appropriate. The nurse may have a good reason for refusing to give the medication and therefore Option H would be an appropriate course of action.

III. You are a FY2 doctor working on a busy surgical ward. During a weekend shift one of the nurses asks to speak with you in confidence. She is concerned about another FY2 doctor Andrew. The nurse tells you that she witnessed Andrew make a number of mistakes today and when she told him this he started crying and said he was struggling to handle his workload.

Choose the **THREE most appropriate** *actions to take in this situation.*

A. Seek advice from senior colleagues about how to support Andrew
B. Suggest the nurse advises Andrew to make an appointment with occupational health
C. Speak to Andrew about the nurse's concerns
D. Talk to your FY2 colleagues about redistributing workload within the team
E. Suggest that the nurse escalates her concerns to your consultant
F. Inform Andrew's clinical supervisor about his difficulties prioritising his

workload
G. Report Andrew to the GMC
H. Do nothing, Andrew is likely going through a difficult time and things will get better

Answers: A, C, D

Option A demonstrates willingness to escalate to a senior colleague and would be appropriate should you feel out of your depth. Option C is likely to be the first option to take in this scenario as a simple conversation with Andrew may unearth the reasons why he is struggling. It is likely that in the short term, in order to maintain patient safety, your other FY2 colleagues will have to take on some of Andrew's tasks (Option D).

IV. During your GP rotation, you are in the waiting area calling a patient through to your consultation room. Your GP supervisor happens to walk past and begins to berate you for ordering the wrong blood tests on a patient you saw earlier in the day.

Choose the **THREE most appropriate** actions to take in this situation.

A. Discuss with the reception staff whether this has happened before
B. Approach your supervisor later in private to suggest that his behaviour was inappropriate
C. Apologise to any patients who may have overheard
D. Take no action as your supervisor is probably having a bad day
E. Document the interaction in your electronic portfolio
F. Review your notes from the previous consultation
G. Berate your supervisor in return, as you feel you should defend yourself in front of your patients
H. Ask another senior GP for advice

Answers: B, C, H

Option B shows that you are dealing with the situation directly and doing so in a private place away from patients. Option C is an important step to take because patients may be alarmed by what they have heard and protecting the doctor-patient relationship and trust in the practice is paramount. Option H would be an appropriate step to take should you feel out of your depth and it may be the case that a more senior GP is better placed to speak with your supervisor.

V. You are the FY2 doctor looking after the medical ward. The wife of a 58-year-old man admitted in acute alcohol withdrawal angrily approaches you claiming you are not doing your job properly and her husband is not getting better.

Choose the **THREE most appropriate** actions to take in this situation.

SRA: 2.2 Professional Dilemas

A. Refuse to answer the wife's questions as she is being abusive
B. Speak to a senior colleague for support
C. Re-assess the patient
D. Call hospital security to remove the wife from the ward
E. Tell the wife that you are about to finish your shift but somebody else will talk to her
F. Submit an incident report
G. Arrange a meeting between the consultant and the patient's wife
H. Record the incident in your electronic portfolio

Answers: B, C, G

Option B would be an appropriate option given that this situation may be beyond your capabilities and a senior colleague may be better placed to deal with it. There may be good reason why the patient's wife is upset and so clinically re-assessing the patient (Option C) ensures that any urgent issues regarding patient safety are identified. Option G is a sensible option as your consultant is likely to know the most about the patient's plan going forward. Arranging a meeting between the two parties may be all that is needed to reassure the wife.

2.3 Clinical Problem Solving (CPS)

This paper consists of 97 questions in 75 minutes. You will be tested on how well you apply clinical judgement and problem solving skills to determine appropriate diagnosis and management of patients. The knowledge tested will be appropriate to the level of a FY2 doctor. Only 86 questions count towards the final score, as 11 questions are for piloting purposes only. The test covers five core competencies:

1. Investigation
2. Diagnosis
3. Emergency
4. Prescribing
5. Management (non-prescribing)

For each question, one mark is awarded for choosing the correct response. For each MBA, multiple marks are awarded for each correct response (up to a maximum of 3 marks). Even if you are unsure, it is always best to attempt to answer the question as there is no negative marking.

Each paper will be given a score and banded 1-4. You will be notified of your score and band for both the PD/SJT paper and the CPS paper via ORIEL. Due to normalisation of all scores, there is no maximum achievable score, however a score of 575 approximately represents the top 10 percentile. In 2016, a minimum score of 354 was required to be considered for an invitation to interview. However, only those candidates scoring 458 and above were invited in the first round. Essentially, the majority of candidates are still invited to interview and so a decent performance will ensure that you make it onto the interview shortlist.

Questions are in three formats:

Extended Matching Questions (EMQs)

Examples

I. Endocrine disorders

A. Acromegaly
B. Diabetes
C. Hyperthyroidism
D. Hypothyroidism
E. Hypoparathyroidism
F. Hypopituitarism

For each patient, what is the **SINGLE** *most likely diagnosis?*
Select **ONE** *option only from the list above. Each option may be selected once, more than once, or not at all.*

SRA: 2.3 Clinical Problem Solving (CPS)

1. A 40-year-old man presents with headaches and joint pains. On examination, he is found to be hypertensive and have a bitemporal hemianopia.
2. A 58-year-old woman presents with generalised fatigue. On further questioning she admits to feeling cold all the time and experiencing tingling in her hand at night.
3. A 15-year old boy presents to A&E feeling drowsy and unwell. Urinalysis reveals the presence of ketones.

Answers: 1A, 2D, 3B

Acromegaly is an excess of growth hormone (GH) and is usually caused by a pituitary tumour. It can present with signs and symptoms caused by the tumour itself (headache, visual defects), or due to excess GH (coarsening of features, sweating, joint pains, hypertension). Hypothyroidism often presents insidiously with tiredness, dry skin, hair loss, constipation, weight gain and reduced libido. Tingling in the hand is caused by carpal tunnel syndrome which is associated with hypothyroidism. Type I diabetes can present in the acute setting as diabetic ketoacidosis (DKA). DKA is a medical emergency characterised by hyperglycaemia, acidosis and ketoneamia. Treatment is with IV insulin, fluids and management of the precipitating cause (if present).

II. Dermatological disorders

A. Acne vulgaris
B. Rosacea
C. Acanthosis nigricans
D. Lupus pernio
E. Sclerodactyly
F. Shagreen patch

For each patient, what is the **SINGLE** *most likely diagnosis?*
Select **ONE** *option only from the list above. Each option may be selected once, more than once, or not at all.*

1. A 5-year-old boy with a history of epilepsy presents with a flesh-coloured patch on his lower back
2. A 75-year old man with advanced gastric malignancy presents with darkened patches of skin in his axilla
3. A 45-year-old woman with known sarcoidosis presents with a painless purple nodule on her nose

Answers: 1F, 2C, 3D

Shagreen patches are a common feature of tuberous sclerosis. Other skin manifestations include angiofibromas, ungual fibromas and ash leaf-shaped white macules. Acanthosis nigricans presents with thickened brown velvety-textured patches within the skin folds including armpit, groin and back of the neck. It is associated with internal malignancy, most commonly stomach cancer. Lupus pernio is associated with sarcoidosis of the lungs and presents as reddish-purple plaques and nodules on the nose, lips, cheeks and ears.

III. Common side-effects

A. Spironolactone
B. Ramipirl
C. Digoxin
D. Bendroflumethiazide
E. Amiodarone
F. Doxazosin

For each presentation, what is the **SINGLE** *most likely cause?*
Select **ONE** *option only from the list above. Each option may be selected once, more than once, or not at all.*

1. A 74-year-old woman presents to her GP with a dry cough
2. An 80-year old man attends the emergency department complaining of an acutely hot and swollen right big toe
3. A 70-year-old woman presents to her GP complaining of seeing a bluish halo in her vision. On examination, her skin is noted to have a blue-grey tinge.

Answers: 1B, 2D, 3E

Ramipril is an ACE inhibitor and commonly causes a dry cough. Other side-effects include angioedema and renal impairment, and kidney function should be monitored after starting treatment. Bendroflumethiazide is a thiazide diuretic which can lead to hyperuricameia and gout. Amiodarone has a number of side-effects including pulmonary fibrosis and thyroid dysfunction. Corneal microdeposits may cause some patients to complain of seeing a bluish halo and skin discoloration may also occur.

IV. A child with a limp

A. Perthes disease
B. Reactive arthritis
C. Slipped upper femoral epiphysis
D. Developmental dysplasia of the hip
E. Transient synovitis
F. Septic arthritis

For each child, what is the **SINGLE** *most likely diagnosis?*
Select **ONE** *option only from the list above. Each option may be selected once, more than once, or not at all.*

1. A 10-year old boy presents with a gradual onset of right-sided hip pain. On examination, he has a limited range of hip movement but is otherwise well.
2. A 3-year old girl with a recent diagnosis of a viral upper respiratory tract infection refuses to walk. On, examination she is febrile and will not allow her hip to be examined.

3. The parents of an 8-week old girl with a history of breech presentation attend the ultrasound department for screening.

Answers: 1A, 2F, 3D

Perthes disease is caused by avascular necrosis of the femoral head and usually presents with a gradual onset of pain and limp. Ongoing management should include an x-ray and prompt orthopaedic referral. Septic arthritis is an orthopaedic emergency and presents as a hot swollen joint in a systemically unwell child. A hip ultrasound may show an effusion and blood tests would reveal a raised WCC and CRP. Treatment is with intravenous antibiotics. Developmental dysplasia of the hip is more common in breech presentations as well as in first-degree relatives of those with the condition. In the UK, there is a national screening programme which involves a hip ultrasound at 6 weeks for those considered to be at high risk.

V. Reproductive health

A. Ruptured ovarian cyst
B. Uterine fibroids
C. Endometriosis
D. Appendicitis
E. Adenomyosis
F. Ectopic pregnancy

For each patient, what is the **SINGLE** *most likely diagnosis?*
Select **ONE** *option only from the list above. Each option may be selected once, more than once, or not at all.*

1. A 28-year old woman presents to the emergency department with acute onset of right iliac fossa pain. She has had her appendix removed during a previous admission. A urine beta-HCG is positive.
2. A 32-year old woman presents to her GP with heavy periods and dyspareunia. She has noticed spotting in between her periods.
3. A 24-year old woman presents to the emergency department with left iliac fossa pain. A urine beta-HCG is negative.

Answers: 1F, 2C, 3A

A ruptured ectopic pregnancy is a gynaecological emergency and presents with sudden onset abdominal or pelvic pain. A pregnancy test should be carried out on all women presenting with abdominal pain in whom pregnancy is a possibility. Endometriosis is the presence of endometrial tissue outside the uterine cavity. Symptoms include dysmenorrhoea, dyspareunia, abdominal pain, infertility and menstrual problems. Ruptured ovarian cysts are one of the most common causes of pain in premenopausal women. A negative pregnancy test helps differentiate it from ectopic pregnancy.

SRA: 2.3 Clinical Problem Solving (CPS)

Multiple Best Answer (MBA)

Examples

I. A 56-year-old man with a history of acute pancreatitis presents to the Emergency Department with abdominal pain and vomiting.

Which **THREE** of the following indicates a poor prognosis in this patient? Select **THREE** options only.

A. Age of 56
B. BP of 95/60
C. Calcium of 1.8 mmol/L
D. Confusion
E. Glucose of 7 mmol/L
F. Respiratory rate of 22 per minute
G. WBC of 18 x 109 /L

Answer: A, C, G

Scoring systems such as the Glasgow score have been shown to increase accuracy of prognosis in acute pancreatitis. Criteria included in the Glasgow scoring system are:

- Age >55 years
- WBC >15 x 109/L
- Urea >16 mmol/L
- Glucose >10 mmol/L
- pO2 <8 kPa (60 mm Hg)
- Albumin <32 g/L
- Calcium <2 mmol/L
- LDH >600 units/L
- AST/ALT >200 units

Other scoring systems include Ranson's criteria, APACHE II and Balthazar.

II. A 28-year-old man presents to his GP complaining of persistent low mood for the last three weeks.

Which **THREE** of the following support a diagnosis of mild depression? Select **THREE** options only.

A. Disturbed sleep
B. Auditory hallucinations
C. Delusions of grandeur
D. Poor appetite
E. Inability to concentrate
F. Visual hallucinations
G. Obsessional thoughts

SRA: 2.3 Clinical Problem Solving (CPS)

Answer: A, D, E

According to ICD-10, the diagnostic criteria for depression include ten depressive symptoms. Key symptoms include: persistent low mood, anhedonia and fatigue. If any of these are present most days for at least two weeks then the following associated symptoms should also be asked about: disturbed sleep, inability to concentrate, low self-confidence, poor or increased appetite, suicidal thoughts, agitation or slowing of movements and feelings of guilt. Mild depression is defined as the presence of four symptoms.

III. A 74-year-old man is seen in cardiology outpatients and is noted to have an ejection systolic murmur radiating to the carotids.

Which **THREE** of the following symptoms is this patient most likely to complain of? Select **THREE** options only.

A. Syncope
B. Paroxysmal nocturnal dyspnoea
C. Angina
D. Exertional dyspnoea
E. Orthopnoea
F. Malar flush
G. Abdominal swelling

Answers: A, C, D

This gentleman has the characteristic murmur of aortic stenosis. A classic triad of 'SAD' is often described: syncope, angina and dyspnoea. Diagnostic investigations include an ECG, blood tests and an echocardiogram. Aortic stenosis is graded according to its severity on echocardiogram and patients with severe or symptomatic disease may be eligible for surgical aortic valve repair.

IV. A 28-year-old patient with a diagnosis of neurofibromatosis type II presents with worsening horizontal diplopia. Examination reveals an isolated abduction palsy of the right eye.

Which **THREE** of the following cranial nerves are responsible for eye movements? Select **THREE** options only.

A. CN II
B. CN III
C. CN IV
D. CN V
E. CN VI
F. CN VII
G. CN IX

Answers: B, C, E

SRA: 2.3 Clinical Problem Solving (CPS)

This patient has neurofibromatosis type II and is therefore at risk of developing an acoustic neuroma which may involve CN VI (abducens) within the cerebellopontine angle. CN VI is responsible for abduction, therefore a mononeuropathy affecting it will result in a horizontal diplopia. Other cranial nerves responsible for eye movements are CN III (oculomotor) and CN IV (trochlear).

V. A 70-year-old man presents to his GP with an increasing frequency of falls. Neurological examination demonstrates 'cog-wheeling'.

Which **THREE** of the following features might you associate with this presentation? Select **THREE** options only.

A. Reduced muscle tone
B. Hyperkineasia
C. Bradykinesia
D. Rigidity
E. Brisk reflexes
F. Resting tremor
G. Cerebellar ataxia

Answers: C, D, F

This gentleman exhibits a characteristic examination finding of Parkinson's disease, caused by a combination of resting tremor and rigidity. Bradykinesia is another feature of Parkinson's disease and presents as a slowness of voluntary movement. This may be demonstrated by reduced arm swinging whilst walking or by a reduced amplitude of repetitive movement (e.g. repeatedly opposing thumb and middle finger).

Single Best Answer (SBA)

Examples

I. A 75-year-old woman develops shortness of breath three days after a total abdominal hysterectomy. Her chest is clear on auscultation, but her left calf appears swollen and tender.

Select the **SINGLE** most likely **diagnosis** from the list below, Select **ONE** option only.

A. Asthma
B. Left ventricular failure
C. Pneumothorax
D. Pulmonary embolus
E. Pulmonary haemorrhage

Answer: D

SRA: 2.3 Clinical Problem Solving (CPS)

The Wells criteria is a risk stratification score used to predict the likelihood of pulmonary embolism (PE). Criteria which make a diagnosis of PE more likely include recent immobilisation or surgery and unilateral calf swelling. Using a two-tier model, patients are categorised as either low or high risk for PE. In conjunction with a negative D-dimer, PE can effectively be ruled out in low risk patients.

II. A 53-year-old Afro-Caribbean man is referred to the cardiology outpatient department due to concerns over his blood pressure. Average readings over a 2-week period are above 160/100 mmHg. Fundoscopy is unremarkable. What is the most suitable management option:

Select the **SINGLE** *most likely* **diagnosis** *from the list below, Select* **ONE** *option only.*

A. Start amlodipine
B. Start bendroflumethiazide
C. Start ramipril
D. No treatment required
E. Continue monitoring blood pressure for another two weeks

Answer: A

According to NICE guidelines, all hypertensive patients aged 55 or over or of Afro-Caribbean descent should be started on a calcium channel blocker. All hypertensive patients below 55 should be started on an angiotensin converting enzyme (ACE) inhibitor or an angiotensin II receptor antagonist.

III. A 33-year-old woman attends the Emergency Department with central chest pain worse on leaning forwards. She describes a history of a recent upper respiratory tract infection. An ECG demonstrates widespread concave ST elevation. What is the most likely diagnosis:

Select the **SINGLE** *most likely* **diagnosis** *from the list below, Select* **ONE** *option only.*

A. Costochondritis
B. Pulmonary embolism
C. Pancreatitis
D. Myocardial infarction
E. Pericarditis

Answer: E

Pericarditis refers to inflammation of the pericardium. Characteristic ECG features include widespread concave or 'saddle-shaped' ST elevation and PR depression. It may be associated with a recent viral illness. Other associations include TB, systemic lupus erythematosus and rheumatoid arthritis. Treatment is with NSAIDs.

IV. A 24-year-old woman presents to her GP complaining of weight gain and irregular periods. On examination you notice facial acne and unusual hair on the upper lip. What is the most likely diagnosis:

Select the **SINGLE** *most likely* **diagnosis** *from the list below, Select* **ONE** *option only.*

A. Hyperthyroidism
B. Hyperprolactinaemia
C. Acromegaly
D. Polycystic ovary syndrome
E. Cushing's syndrome

Answer: D

Polycystic ovary syndrome presents classically with symptoms including oligomenorrhoea, acne, hirsutism, obesity and low mood. Diagnostic tests include total or free testosterone levels, LH:FSH ratio and ovarian ultrasound demonstrating the presence of polycystic ovaries.

V. An 85-year-old man presents to his GP complaining of exertional breathlessness. He reports a history of rheumatic fever as a child. On examination, there is a low-pitched diastolic murmur heard loudest at the apex. What is the most likely diagnosis?

Select the **SINGLE** *most likely* **diagnosis** *from the list below, Select* **ONE** *option only.*

A. Aortic stenosis
B. Mitral regurgitation
C. Tricuspid regurgitation
D. Mitral stenosis
E. Pulmonary stenosis

Answer: D

Symptoms of mitral stenosis include breathlessness, orthopnoea and paroxysmal nocturnal dyspnoea. The characteristic murmur is a low-pitched rumbling diastolic murmur heard loudest over the apex. Mitral stenosis is strongly associated with rheumatic fever, however this an increasingly less common cause in the developed world. Other clinical signs include a raised jugular venous pressure or a malar flush. Aortic regurgitation is another diastolic murmur heard loudest over the left sternal border.

3 PORTFOLIO STATION

3.1 Specific questions **60**
   3.1.1 Clinical radiology experience 60
   3.1.2 Audit 62
   3.1.3 Teaching 64
   3.1.4 Exams 66
   3.1.5 Research 67

3.2 Motivational questions. **69**
   3.2.1 What is your proudest achievement? 69
   3.2.2 What is your greatest strength? 70
   3.2.3 What is your main weakness? 71

3.3 Situational ability questions **74**
   3.3.1 Communication skills 74
   3.3.2 Risk management 75
   3.3.3 Problem Solving 77
   3.3.4 Empathy 78
   3.3.5 Team work 80
   3.3.6 Time management 81
   3.3.7 Judgment 82
   3.3.8 Leadership 83
   3.3.9 Conflict resolution 85
   3.3.10 Probity 86

3.1 Specific Questions

3.1.1 Clinical radiology experience

Question
- Take me through your CV

Alternative questions
- Tell me about yourself.
- Why should you be offered a radiology training number?

What the interviewers are looking for

During the portfolio station, the interviewers go through the candidates' self-assessment of their portfolios and ensure they have marked themselves fairly by reviewing evidence of their achievements. The questions tend to be on more specific areas like teaching, audit or evidence of reflection. It is however more than possible that candidates may be asked to summarise their CV/portfolio. It is your chance to shine, so use the question as an opportunity to demonstrate your achievements to the interviewers.

How to answer

The CAMP framework is very helpful for general background questions like this and we would advise using it so that your answer retains a structure and focus.

Approach

Clinical	• Briefly summarise your career with a focus on how this has prepared you for training in radiology. Mention taster weeks as these will score you points.
Academic	• Degrees and exams • Teaching, teaching courses and qualifications • Audits and research you have completed
Management	• Leadership roles and committees you have been part of • Courses you have organised • Guidelines you have written
Personal	• Personal skills that you have • Interests and hobbies

Example

"My name is John Smith and I am currently a FY2 Doctor at St Alexander's Hospital in London. I have had a broad range of clinical experience in the Foundation Programme with rotations through several medical and surgical specialties. Cardiology and vascular surgery were particularly useful rotations because of the practical skills

I developed such as placing central lines. During my taster week I was therefore able to assist during some interventional radiology sessions and got more out of it as a result. Also, the busy nature of these rotations meant that I quickly learnt to prioritise my work based on clinical urgency – a skill I noted during my taster week to be vital during busy on-calls as a radiology trainee.

I thoroughly enjoy teaching and have been involved in teaching medical students locally on chest and abdominal radiographs. I also organised a national medical finals revision course. Through working with a group of seven Foundation trainees in organising this, I developed leadership and team working skills. The course was a success with over 90% of students feeling more confident about finals after undertaking the course. Completion of Part 1 of the MRCP has further helped develop my medical knowledge and will form a platform to prepare for the challenging FRCR exams in the future. I recently led an audit on assessing the appropriateness of abdominal radiographs. As a result of the interventions I made, there has been a 50% reduction in the number of films performed with over 90% fitting the highlighted indications. As the Foundation trainee representative, I have helped resolve local issues like trainees not being able to attend teaching and have developed negotiating and problem solving skills as a result. My multisource feedback shows that my colleagues feel I am dependable, well organised and a good communicator who works towards ensuring the best possible outcome for patients. Outside of medicine, I am a keen, albeit variably successful, football and squash player and I enjoy travelling and reading."

TOP TIPS

➕ **Selling Yourself:** This can often prove challenging as candidates do not wish to come off as overconfident or cocky. Rather use examples and feedback to demonstrate how good you are e.g. 'My 360-degree appraisal graded my communication skills as excellent'

➕ **Be Positive and Sell, Sell, Sell:** Interviewers want to hear how great you are and it is important that you are not bashful or reserved when telling them about your achievements and why they should choose you. Turn everything into a positive and don't undersell yourself.

3.1.2 Audit

Question
- Tell me about your best audit.

Alternative questions
- What makes a good audit?
- What is your experience of audit / what audits have you completed?

What the interviewers are looking for

Audit plays a vital role in all medical specialties and radiology is no exception. Audit or quality improvement projects have been included in the radiology interviews in some capacity or another for many years now. The interviewers are ideally looking for you to have played a key role in a radiology-relevant audit that focused on patient safety and clinical improvement, which ideally changed practice for the better.

How to answer

Even if not specifically asked, it is always important to use an example when answering a question about audit. Talking about just one good one in more depth, including your role, how it benefited practice and what you learnt will impress the interviewers more than listing lots of audits and not expanding on them.

To pick a good audit, it is important that you have a succinct definition of audit and are extremely familiar with the well-recognised 'audit cycle'. The Healthcare Quality Improvement Partnership (HQIP) definition is stated below. HQIP also provide a helpful summary of the audit cycle in their document, 'Best Practice in Clinical Audit' that is available online.

"Clinical audit is a quality improvement cycle that involves measurement of the effectiveness of healthcare against agreed and proven standards for high quality, and taking action to bring practice in line with these standards so as to improve the quality of care and health outcomes."

Make sure you stress how important your role in the audit was. If asked about your "best" or "most interesting" audit, pick the audit that covers as many of the important points indicated above (radiology-relevant, changed practice, patient safety etc.) even if you don't necessarily think it is the most interesting thing you have ever done. It is also important that you know the key results from the audits included in your portfolio.

Approach

Using the components of the audit cycle provides a clear framework for structuring your answer and clearly indicates that you understand the audit cycle. These are namely:

Stage 1: Identifying a problem or issue
Stage 2: Identifying a standard
Stage 3: Data collection
Stage 4: Comparing current performance against the standard
Stage 5: Implementing change
Stage 6: Re-audit ('closing the loop')

Example

"The most interesting audit I have completed was one that I designed and led and which resulted in a direct improvement to patient care. I noticed during my taster week that a large number of patients who were scheduled for CT-guided biopsies of suspected lung cancers were cancelled due to the frequent lack of patient beds on the ward where the patients went for observation after the procedure. I decided to audit the cancellation rate over two months with the agreed standard that ideally no patients should have their biopsy cancelled purely due to the lack of a bed when a cancer diagnosis was suspected. During the two months, 25% of biopsies were cancelled due to a lack of beds, resulting in an average delay of five days before the biopsies were rescheduled. I used my initiative and problem solving skills to identify beds that were often not in full use in the nearby endoscopy recovery ward. The respiratory specialist nurse, my supervisor and I trained the endoscopy recovery nurses regarding the specific post-lung biopsy care instructions. Patients now head to endoscopy for recovery after lung biopsies. Just 5% of cases were cancelled during a two-month re-audit and 20% more biopsies were performed during the same time period. I estimated this also saved the trust around £3000 over two months due to reduced inpatient occupancy and all but one patient went home the same day without significant complication. I am grateful for the opportunity to have completed this audit and developed team working, problem solving and leadership skills as a result."

TOP TIPS

 Audit Summary. It is a good idea to create a single A4 sheet summarising each of your audit projects using the subheadings above. This has two purposes: to remind you of the key points and facts of each audit and to make the audits easier to find within your portfolio.

3.1.3 Teaching

Question:
- Tell us about your teaching experience.

Alternative questions
- What makes a good teacher?
- What kind of teaching methods do you know?
- Why is teaching important?

What the interviewers are looking for

Teaching is a very common theme at radiology interviews. There is sure to be a significant number of points ascribed to teaching. The interviewers ideally want to see evidence of the use of several teaching methods, participation in teaching courses and evidence of teaching feedback with reflection on how the feedback has altered your practice.

How to answer

In order to demonstrate a broad range of teaching experience, you should structure your answer into the different types of teaching methods you have used, together with succinct summaries of specific examples. You also need to mention feedback and highlight examples in your portfolio. It is ok and encouraged to mention good feedback, but also select some feedback that indicates an area for improvement and explain how you have acted upon this. Discussing any teaching courses you have been on and what you learnt will further strengthen your answer. Finally, finishing with some thoughts on why you enjoy teaching and indicating some of the other personal skills it allows you to develop should help you to reach a natural conclusion.

As indicated, another common variation of the question would be to talk about the qualities of a good teacher so reflect on this before the interview. Some good qualities include:

- Clear communicator and well organised
- Adaptable to the needs of the students
- Involves the students heavily in their own learning – teasing ideas out and encouraging students to make their own realisations helps take learning to a deeper level of understanding
- Employs several methods of teaching
- Gathers and acts on feedback

Approach

Break your answer down into:

1. Teaching methods you have used, with examples
2. Discuss feedback and what you have learnt

Portfolio: 3.1.3 Teaching

3. Any teaching courses you have been on and what you learnt
4. Why you enjoy teaching and the skills it has helped you to develop

Example: CV weakness

"I have thoroughly enjoyed teaching throughout my career to date and have employed several teaching methods. During my Foundation years, I have regularly taught medical students on the wards on an informal basis. This has taught me to be adaptable, but I have also learnt that highlighting a specific area for each student to focus on before the teaching ensures that there is a structure and clear goals for each student. I have also organised more formal, didactic teaching in the form of a series of lectures to medical students on chest, abdominal and trauma radiographs at my local hospital. I made use of a quiz and encouraged questions and discussions to ensure that the lectures remained interactive. I always gather feedback from any teaching I give to ensure I make further improvements next time. I was delighted that over 90% of students felt more comfortable interpreting plain films after my lectures, but it was this comment that I found the most useful, "excellent example images, but please include more clinical history/information on management as we are still learning these." I now try and do this with every medical student teaching session and have received some positive feedback regarding this already. I have been on several teaching courses to help further develop my teaching skills. One that was particularly useful was on problem based learning at the local University. I had not taught or been taught with this method before, but can now see one big advantage in that by encouraging students to make their own discoveries, a deeper, more thorough level of understanding can be achieved and I will make use of this particular point in my future practice. As well as enjoying the teaching itself, I am grateful that it has allowed me to develop several other transferrable skills such as organisational skills in planning sessions and problem solving when helping with specific questions. I look forward to continuing to teach and develop further in the future."

TOP TIP

 Feedback. Always remember to include written feedback in your portfolio. If you can't show the interviewers your teaching feedback it's hard for them to award you points.

3.1.4 Exams

Question
- Tell us about any postgraduate exams you have completed.

Alternative questions
- Radiology is an exam-heavy specialty. How have you demonstrated your commitment to study for these?

What the interviewers are looking for

Again, if recent years' interviews are anything to go by, this is likely to be more of a tick box exercise. The interviewers are looking for evidence of completion of postgraduate examinations commensurate with your level of training so make sure you highlight these and show evidence if asked.

How to answer

This may well just be a tick box answer, but if you do have to discuss this in more detail, then think about what you learnt, how the exam(s) was/were useful for radiology and whether you are planning to take any more.

Example

"I completed the MRCS Part A examination two thirds of the way through my FY1 year and am currently studying to sit the Part B examination in October. I learnt from my taster week, that the best radiologists have an excellent foundation in both medicine and surgery, they are aware of how imaging fits into the workup of particular presentations and can therefore produce clinically helpful reports that benefit the patient. Studying for these postgraduate examinations has helped developed my knowledge of a range of pathologies and their management. I am also hoping that the development of my understanding of anatomy will help both with my FRCR Part 1 anatomy exam as well as in my future career in general. Finally, balancing studying for these exams with working busy rotations and trying to maintain a social life has taught me the importance of remaining organised and to plan well in advance in order to efficiently manage my time."

3.1.5 Research

- Tell us about your research experience.

Alternative questions
- Is research important / should all radiology trainees do research?
- What is the difference between research and audit?
- How would you critically analyse a paper/research project?

What the interviewers are looking for

Understandably, candidates' research experience will vary greatly depending on their career path to date and the interviewers will understand this. They are primarily looking for an understanding of research principles and the ethical issues of research, as well as evidence of completion of research in the form of publications, intercalated degrees or possibly further postgraduate degrees.

How to answer

As with audit questions, it is important to talk about the specifics of any research you have done. Creating a summary about each project and placing it in your portfolio will help you to succinctly summarise your research. How you answer the question depends on your research experience. If you haven't done much research, then talking about literature reviews you have done can be helpful to show that you are well aware of the principles of research, how to do it and how to critically analyse it. If you have got a few publications, you can talk about one or two of those projects in more detail, as well as summarising your research experience e.g., "I have completed my BSc/PhD in XX, authored XX papers and done XX international presentations, but the project I am most proud of is XX."

As with any question about your experience of something, it is vital to state what you learnt from doing it and this should include generic, transferrable skills such as leadership and team working (see the 'Personal Skills' section of the person specification). You should also mention any research orientated courses you have attended (and what you learnt) as well as any funding you have secured – whether that be for research or things like elective bursaries, as that still shows that you have the ability to write a successful grant application.

Whilst not everyone has to do it, make sure you are aware of the importance of research and can distinguish between research and audit.

Approach

When describing a research project, use a logical structure similar to what you would use when writing an abstract (background, method, results etc.), but also state what you learnt, including knowledge of research principles and also generic, personal skills. If you haven't completed any research yet you can talk about the methodology of any project you are currently undertaking in more detail. Also mention grants/bursaries you have gained and any research courses you have completed.

Example

 "My research experience started with my intercalated degree in physiology for which I achieved a first class honours and I have since been the first author of three published research papers. The project I am most proud of however is one I completed as part of my elective. To give some background, patients respond to angioplasty for claudication differently and it can be difficult to establish who will or won't benefit. I gained ethical approval to conduct a study and personally recruited 20 patients in which I took blood before, immediately after and 6 weeks after angioplasty for claudication. With the help of a research team, we analysed these samples using a technique called metabonomics and identified a metabolite that was associated with a favourable response to angioplasty. I concluded that this could be a marker for predicating a positive response to angioplasty, but would need further validation. I am particularly proud of it because I applied and further developed skills I had learnt at the undergraduate level to an actual research project, namely writing a successful ethics application, consenting patients for research and analysing data to against a null hypothesis. I also felt my critical analysis skills have improved, because with the help of my supervisors, I reached a fair and sensible conclusion that recognised the need for further validation. I also completed a 'Good Ethical Practice' research course at my university, before doing this project and successfully gained £2000 in funding from a research grant. Whilst I have completed one radiology research project about an iterative reconstruction technique for CT KUB studies, I am looking forward to further applying and developing my research methodology skills in my chosen career of radiology."

TOP TIPS

➕ **Selling Yourself.** This can often prove challenging as candidates do not wish to come off as overconfident or cocky. Rather use examples and feedback to demonstrate how good you are.

➕ **Be Specific.** Similar to the audit section above make sure that you know all the facts and figures related to your research.

3.2 Motivational Questions

3.2.1 What is your proudest achievement?

Alternative questions
- What is your proudest achievement outside of medicine?

What the interviewers are looking for

A memorable, clearly significant achievement that stands you out from your peers and ideally demonstrates you to be a balanced individual. The interviewers also want to see evidence of reflection on the event and how it will make you a good person to work with and a better radiologist.

How to answer

This question may have caught some people by surprise at last year's interviews, but the person specification does specifically mention, "evidence of achievement outside of medicine." With this in mind, it is well worth considering using a non-medically related example. If a non-academic achievement is not specified and there is an academic achievement you haven't mentioned and you really are proud of it, you could consider asking the interviewer whether they meant medical or non-medical. Try to avoid mentioning more than one as you are not answering the question and you may dilute each answer's strengths. Either way, you need to emphasise the significance and describe what you learnt from the achievement.

Approach

If choosing a medical example think of the CAM of CAMP. The P of CAMP covers some of the non-medical examples. Consider achievements related to your hobbies or extracurricular activities at university. The person specification includes, "evidence of altruistic behaviour...and organisation skills," so voluntary work you have done or achievements related to organisational roles should also be considered. When selecting your achievement, consider how many other candidates are likely to have done the same thing. It does not have to be truly unique, but you shouldn't choose something everyone will have done.

The basic approach is to explain it, explain the significance of it and what you learnt.

Example

"My biggest achievement to date is when I was at medical school in my 4th year I personally organised a dance show involving over 150 students, with an audience of 2000 people that raised over £15,000 for a children's cancer charity.   I am particularly proud of this primarily because of the amount of money *that it raised for such a wonderful cause. Furthermore, it was a privilege to work with all the committee members and dancers to organise a very well received show. Not only was it an enjoyable experience, but also one I learnt a lot from. Fourth year was our toughest year in terms of exams, so in order to ensure that organising the show did not compromise my studies, I planned both well in advance to ensure I could allocate enough time to both and I feel my organisation and prioritisation skills have improved as a result. I believe this will help me both outside of medicine and (hopefully!) in a radiology career in the future."*

TOP TIPS

 Reflect. Remember that points are awarded for why the achievement is so special and how it relates to radiology. Make sure you reflect on the underlying skills and values and try to use the person specification to relate back to radiology.

3.2.2 What is your greatest strength?

Alternative questions
- What is the strongest area of your CV?
- What makes you stand out against other applicants?

What the interviewers are looking for

The interviewers want to know your key selling points that make you suitable for a radiology training post. They want to establish whether your strengths are compatible with a career in radiology and gain insight into your character and self-confidence.

How to answer

The key is not to recite a list of desirable characteristics, but to select a few that you consider to be the strongest areas of your CV. Use actual examples from your training thus far to demonstrate these strengths and reflect on how they relate to radiology training. Medics are notoriously bad at selling themselves and often worry that talking about their achievements will come across as over-confident. Whilst this should not be the aim, under-selling your achievements is equally as detrimental.

Approach

This question can be approached using CAMP, or more simply by using one clinical and one extracurricular achievement. Beyond two examples and you risk running out of time for subsequent questions.

Clinical	Extracurricular
Publication	Marathon
Organising a conference	Team sports
Updating guidelines	Playing a musical instrument
Postgraduate exams	Charity work
Teaching	

Example

"I have many strengths which are evidenced by my excellent 360-degree feedback from colleagues and peers. However, the two areas which I consider to be my greatest strengths are my teaching skills and my organisational skills. I have demonstrated both of these when I organised an emergency radiology course for Foundation doctors. This required me to locate a venue, arrange speakers, set a programme for the day and teach on the chest x-ray station. Thirty foundation doctors attended the teaching day and provided unanimously positive feedback. This experience will prove invaluable when teaching juniors and when organising my time between gaining clinical radiology experience and improving my CV during radiology training".

3.2.3 What is your main weakness?

Alternative questions
- What personal skills are you trying to improve on?
- Give an example of a time when your team working / communication / organisation skills could have been better.

What interviewers are looking for

Nobody is perfect and you are not supposed to be the finished article. The interviewers want to see have integrity and want to ensure you have insight into your own abilities. They also want to ensure you reflect on your performance and you try to improve where possible based on events that occur and feedback.

How to answer

You could choose a personal skill or area of your CV. Given the extensive list of personal skills on the person specification and the fact that there is a great deal of scope for reflection on and improvement of personal skills, it makes sense to choose a personal skill. A weak area of your CV is something that could be fairly easily corrected with time.

It is important to choose something you can genuinely relate to and can provide a personal example of. It is also important that that the weakness can also be seen in a positive light and that you explain how you are working to improve it. A reference to its relevance to radiology is also advised.

Approach

- Explain the weakness with a positive slant
- Provide a specific example
- Reflect on it and describe how you are trying to improve it

Example

 "I enjoy working in a team and I also place very high standards on myself. At medical school and whilst working as a Foundation doctor, I have realised that occasionally, when working as part of a team, I can find it frustrating if someone doesn't do something the way I would have done it. A recent example is when I was arranging some medical student teaching with another Foundation doctor, I wanted to predominantly use small group seminars with interactive involvement. The other doctor thought we should just do bedside teaching, which I felt would be inefficient and time consuming. Following discussion, we used my suggestion which resulted in generally good feedback, however there were several comments from students wanting bedside teaching examples to reinforce their knowledge. Based on this feedback, we are subsequently planning to employ both techniques for the next batch of students. This episode made me realise that I need to encourage group discussion when problem solving as part of a team, and listen to other people's suggestions. I am learning that a good team player is flexible and can compromise. I am working hard to ensure I develop these attributes in the future for the good of the team."

TOP TIPS

➕ **Choosing a Weakness.** Don't choose anything too bad, rather select something that is relatable and can be improved

➕ **Don't Dwell On It.** Touch briefly on the weakness and then quickly move the interview towards more positive things

➕ **Identification and Initiative.** Points will be awarded for both identifying a weakness and then demonstrating that you have used your initiative and done something to remedy or improve that weakness. Examples might include finding a mentor, undertaking an audit or research project, attending a course or simply reading up on a topic.

➕ **Follow On Questions.** Be prepared for interviewers to push you for more areas of weakness. One candidate was asked for four further examples of areas that could be improved!

3.3 Situational Ability Questions

3.3.1 Communication skills

Question

Radiologists sit in dark rooms and report scans – do they need good communications skills?

Alternative questions
- Tell us about your communication skills.
- What makes good communication skills?

What the interviewers are looking for

That you have excellent spoken and written communication skills and appreciate why these are important in radiology.

How to answer

The job of a diagnostic radiologist is to interpret imaging and make decisions which benefit patient care. In order to do this, they must produce clear reports for the clinicians – a process which requires excellent written communication skills. Verbal communication skills are also vital because radiologists have direct contact with patients in ultrasound, fluoroscopy and intervention. Excellent verbal communication skills are also important when interacting and negotiating with clinicians during the process of vetting scans, in communicating with them regarding urgent findings and in the setting of multidisciplinary team meetings, where the radiologist plays a key role.

Use personal examples of your own written and verbal communication skills and demonstrate that you know the importance of these in radiology. Excellent communication skills require listening, negotiation and conveying information in a clear, structured way whilst adapting to the setting.

Approach

Use personal examples to demonstrate excellent spoken and written communication skills and acknowledge the important components of good communication skills. Indicate the importance of these skills in radiology.

Example

 "Radiologists certainly do require excellent communication skills and they are somewhat unique in the medical profession in that they must attain excellent written communication skills, as well as verbal ones. This is to convey imaging findings clearly and succinctly with the aim of benefitting patient care. I believe I have developed excellent communication skills through my training so far.

I was very helpfully advised by one of the radiology consultants on my taster week to begin reflecting on the radiology reports that I found most helpful as a clinician. I find that those reports which are structured, succinct and which read well without spelling mistakes give the clearest picture and allow me and my seniors to make the correct management decisions for the patient. Through reflecting on this and with the extensive feedback I have received in achieving several peer-reviewed publications, I believe I have strong written communication skills, which will form the basis for developing my own reporting style in radiology. In terms of verbal communication skills, I would like to use a recent example from my clinical practice. During my current respiratory rotation we had a very unwell 78-year-old patient with severe pneumonia who required transfer to the intensive care unit. My registrar was busy with another sick patient and asked me to make the referral to intensive care. After ensuring I was prepared for the discussion with the relevant information and employing a structured 'SBAR' approach to the referral for clarity, the intensive care registrar was initially reluctant to accept the patient due to their nearly full capacity and our patient's age. I ensured that I actively listened to their concerns and acknowledged their points, but calmly and diplomatically explained why our patient needed intensive care admission and managed to successfully negotiate their admission. I believe my attention to preparation and clear, non-inflammatory method of communication and negotiation will ensure productive discussions with clinicians in the future when I hope to be working as a radiology trainee."

3.3.2 Risk Management

Question

Have you been involved in risk management?

Alternative questions

What do you do to develop/maintain patient safety?

What the interviewers are looking for

That during your clinical practice you maximise patient safety and minimise risk.

How to answer

This may seem a slightly vague question and needs some understanding of what the interviewers are getting at. Medical interviews have moved away from

Portfolio: 3.3.2 Risk Management

candidates having to recite the seven pillars of clinical governance and now focus on competency-based questions with personal answers. Risk management is however one of the traditional pillars of clinical governance and is specifically mentioned on the radiology person specification.

It can be thought of as a process of assessing risks and trying to reduce or minimise them with the aim of optimising safety for patients and staff. It has a pre-emptive focus, but it also recognises that it is vital to learn from mistakes when they do occur in order to minimise future risk.

Personal examples you could use include things like conducting audits, reporting incidents and ensuring lessons are learnt from them, demonstrating evidence of reflection after a mistake and actively supporting your junior colleagues on-call to encourage a culture where people can ask for help.

Approach

Briefly define risk management, before listing specific examples of how you are involved in it.

Example

"Risk management is the systematic process of assessing risk to patients and staff with the aim of minimising these risks. Hospital trusts should have formal policies to do this, but I employ risk management on a daily basis during my clinical practice. In an ideal world, risk management should have a pre-emptive focus. I recently carried out a patient safety focused audit in which I audited the thoracic level that CT KUB scans start at. The radiation dose of all 100 scans fell beneath the national diagnostic reference level, but there was scope for improvement as we noticed many scans included unnecessary imaging of the lower chest and upper abdomen. By commencing the scans at the T10 level, on the re-audit scans remained diagnostic, but the mean dose was reduced by 10%.However, some degree of risk and harm is almost inevitable in healthcare and we must ensure that every possible lesson is learnt when mistakes do occur to try to minimise their reoccurence. During a recent on-call, my junior colleague incorrectly interpreted a difficult, rotated chest radiograph as safe for NG tube feeding, when in fact the tube was in the patient's right lung. As the senior doctor on-call I was asked to review the patient after they became unwell and I instigated the necessary immediate management. Fortunately the patient was unharmed and I offered an apology to them and their family. I was also supportive of the junior and encouraged them to report the incident. I ensured that they felt supported so that they could reflect on what went wrong and encourage them to ask for help in the future. As a result of this event, we organised teaching for all the junior doctors. Because of the blame-free culture we had fostered, the doctor who had misinterpreted the *film felt able to present the case and the learning points to their colleagues. This should maximise safety for patents in the future."*

3.3.3　Problem Solving

Question
Give an example of a time you used problem solving skills to settle an issue at work

Alternative questions
• What is your approach to problem solving?

What the interviewers are looking for

That you demonstrate the ability to think clearly and logically about problems and use an analytical approach efficiently solve them.

How to answer

Radiologists are constantly required to problem solve. This is best done by thoroughly analysing the problem and thinking critically about it with a view to coming up with a solution. You also need to think laterally and come up with suggestions that have not been considered by other members of the clinical team. These skills can be applied to the reporting of a scan, but also to dealing with a busy on-call where you have multiple requests to deal with at once. Use a personal example to demonstrate these skills and illustrate that you understand their importance to radiology.

Approach

When asked to discuss a specific example of when you demonstrated a particular skill, we advise you to use the STAR approach:

- Situation – Briefly set the scene with minimal clinical information as this is not relevant
- Task – Describe the problem you had to solve
- Action – What you personally did and how you went about doing it. Speak in the first person for emphasis
- Result/reflection – State what your hard work achieved and what you learnt

Example

 "I approach problem solving by conducting a critical analysis of all the available information to come up with a rational solution. To give

a recent example, as the Foundation Programme trainee representative, I was asked to draft a medical rota compliant with the new junior doctor contract. Rota-designing is not something I had done before. I set about the task by immediately ensuring I understood the new contract, by thoroughly analysing it and asking for help from the BMA for advice regarding areas I was unsure about. In terms of designing the rota, I spoke to senior trainees and consultants who did have experience of rota-design. I learnt of several unexpected problems they had experienced, such as how to include less than full time trainees. I also sought the thoughts of the junior doctors and medical students who would be working on this contract by sending out a survey. I learnt the two key issues for them were protecting training time and adequate rest. With the wealth of information I had gathered, I designed three different potential rotas and highlighted the relative strengths and weaknesses of each one. I was then able to present these to the medical students and junior doctors who could make informed decisions on a rota that would also be acceptable for hospital management. From the initial feedback, the doctors are happy with the level of training and amount of rest they are now receiving. However, like with any thorough problem solving process, I accept that adjustments may potentially need to be made if any problems are highlighted. I learnt from my taster week that radiologists are constantly required to problem solve, whether they are reporting a tricky scan or managing a busy on call. I believe the analytical methods I have developed will be form a strong starting point from which I can further develop my problem solving skills in the field of radiology."

3.3.4 Empathy

Question
Give an example of where you demonstrated empathy towards a patient

Alternative questions
- Do radiologists need to be sympathetic / empathic?

What the interviewers are looking for

That you are able to take in the perspectives of patients and that you treat them with care and respect. This also applies to your colleagues. There is of course some crossover with questions on communication skills here and you should highlight excellent communication skills as well.

How to answer

It is a lazy criticism of radiology that you lose all patient contact and the skills that go with interacting with patients. If you imply this misconception at interview, it is unlikely to go very well! From the authors' personal experiences, patients who come down to the radiology department for scans are often some of the most complex patients who have often not been informed about what is happening to them. They can be confused or scared as a result, so it is vitally important that radiologists demonstrate the empathy to be aware of this and help reassure them and explain to them what is happening.

Give a personal example of demonstrating empathy, whereby your skills, including communication skills, resulted in a beneficial outcome. Illustrate that you know the importance of this in radiology by highlighting our point in the paragraph above.

Approach

Use the STAR approach as you are asked to demonstrate a skill and the interviewers will be looking for an example.

Example

"During my emergency medicine placement I looked after a young lady who presented with abdominal pain. She had had a few similar presentations over the preceding months with normal observations and blood tests and had been discharged home each time. I sensed that there was an underlying issue, as she seemed tense and scared. In order to explore things further, I suggested that we go to the clinic room which was quieter than the main department. I sensed she wanted to tell me more information and I used open questions and non-verbal communication to encourage her to open up. The poor lady broke down in tears and explained to me that she was feeling so low that she did not know what to do. She didn't want to "trouble" her friends or family and had thought about harming herself. I ensured she had tissues and commended her on speaking out, but also employed moments of silence which helped her open up more. The result was that she was happy to see the liaison psychiatry team who helped create a safe plan for her to be supported in the community.   On reflection, I was happy that having the awareness that something was not right with this lady and encouraging her to speak out in the correct environment meant that she got the help that she needed. From my taster week in radiology, I learnt that importance of empathy and excellent communication skills, as patients often arrive to an alien environment for their ultrasounds or fluoroscopic studies totally uniformed as to why they are there. The radiologist is therefore in the unique position to make a great difference to patients, by listening to their concerns *and help reassuring them. It would be a privilege to able to do this as a radiology trainee and I feel I am developing the skills to do so."*

3.3.5 Team work

Question
Give us an example of a time you displayed good team working skills.

Alternative questions
- Are you a good team player?
- What makes a good team or team player?

What the interviewers are looking for

It is vital that radiologists are good team workers – every day they work with other radiologists, radiographers, radiology department assistants and a variety of clinicians. The interviewers therefore want to ensure you know that you have excellent team working skills and you know what makes a good team.

How to answer

Use a recent example that displays several qualities of good team work and ensure you reflect on the situation. A good team player communicates clearly and effectively, knows their role in the team, knows their own limitations, listens to and respects others and is flexible and adaptable. Explain how these skills you have developed will help in a future career in radiology.

Approach

Use the STAR approach as you are asked to demonstrate a skill and the interviewers will be looking for an example.

Example

""During my current FY2 rotation in haematology I was asked to cover a FY1 teaching session on haematological emergencies by my consultant as he could no longer make the session. Whilst I had gained a lot of experience on-call and felt I could cover much of the basics, I was aware of my own limitations and that I would not be able to cover the whole topic on my own. In order to help the team, I told my consultant that I would be happy to do the teaching, but I asked for some senior help before and during the actual session. I enlisted the help of a senior registrar and whilst I led the teaching session, they added clarification on the more complicated issues when needed. The feedback I received was very positive as I can demonstrate in my portfolio. On reflection, I am glad that I didn't just blindly agree to leading the session without help, as this would have resulted in a poor outcome for the students. The experience reinforced to me the

importance of being aware of one's own limitations and asking for help early when working in a team, to achieve the best possible outcome. From my taster week, I learnt that junior radiology registrars frequently interact with more senior doctors. In order to achieve the best possible outcomes for patients, it will be important to make use of the team, by first listening to the clinicians' concerns, but asking for help early from radiology colleagues when needed."

3.3.6 Time management

Question
How do you organise your workload?

Alternative questions
- How do you manage your time effectively?
- Is it important be organised in radiology? Are you organised?

What the interviewers are looking for

That you demonstrate the ability to manage your time effectively and prioritise tasks appropriately based on clinical need. You should also demonstrate basic professional attributes such as punctuality and reliability.

How to answer

You should use specific examples of how you organise your workload in your clinical practice currently and highlight that you are aware of the transferability of these skills to radiology. Mentioning specific feedback about your organisational skills or reliability will help provide concrete evidence of them.

Approach

Use two or three examples of how you organise your workload and acknowledge the importance of planning and being organised in radiology.

Example

""A recurring theme from my multisource feedback is that my colleagues value my reliability and organisational skills. I employ several methods to organise my workload:

Firstly, it is important to have a record of the tasks in hand. I like to keep our patient list regularly updated so that the team are aware of what needs to be done. With accurate records, it becomes much easier to order the tasks based on clinical priority and delegate the workload appropriately. It also helps highlight those tasks that require undertaking sooner because they take longer, such as organising imaging, so the results are back with sufficient time to safely act on.

Whilst this process is relatively dynamic and alters as clinical priorities change, it is also important to have a degree of fixed structure. To give an example, on vascular surgery we currently have our MDTM on Friday. I therefore ensure that there is a blocked-out period on Thursday morning to ensure we have time to prepare the slides for the meeting. This allows us call for help from other teams much earlier, so that we can meet our emergency ward commitments as well as organise the MDTM.

Finally, whilst I feel I am very organised, it is impossible to prepare for everything, and when I am organising the workload for the day, I ensure we have enough time and hands to account for an emergency should one arise. Having this slack helps us to remain an effective team. I spent some time with the on-call radiology registrar on a Saturday morning to see what it was like and how they coped. I noticed that by keeping a list on the computer updated of all the scans they had agreed to do, they were able to prioritise the most urgent scans and even call down some more routine scans from the ward when it was quieter. Again, it is important to keep some slack as it is only a matter of time before the next emergency scan is needed from A&E and very quickly things can get busy again."

3.3.7 Judgment

Question
Can you work under pressure?

Alternative questions
- How do you deal with uncertainty?
- How do you cope with stress?

What the interviewers are looking for:

The interviewers want the candidate to demonstrate with specific examples that they can work well and efficiently under pressure with the goal of delivering excellent and safe patient care.

How to answer

Use a personal example of a high-pressure situation. Identify that you recognised the pressure, explain how you coped with it, describe what the outcome and what you learned from the experience. Your example should demonstrate initiative, problem solving skills and the ability to ask for help to show that you act safely when under pressure. Try and apply your example to how it will help you in a future career in radiology.

Approach

Use the STAR approach as you are asked to demonstrate a skill and the interviewers will be looking for an example.

Example

 ""I believe I can work under pressure and can use a recent example to demonstrate this. During an on-call in my orthopaedics job I was required to cover the trauma HDU ward due to staff sickness. I was taking referrals for orthopaedics and having to look after sick trauma patients whilst supervising the FY1 on the orthopaedics ward with my registrar busy in theatre. I quickly realised that in the interests of patient safety we would need help so I alerted the on-call orthopaedics consultant who would come in to relieve the registrar from theatre. I also contacted the site practitioner who could help with some ward-based tasks like placing cannulas. With this help, I was able to prioritise reviewing the sickest trauma patients first and identify those who needed early senior input. I was also able to ensure the FY1 was supported with their tasks on the ward. It was a busy day but I could reflect on it with my supervisor the week after. I learnt of the importance of asking for help early, delegating appropriately and prioritising the workload based on clinical need. I believe this will help me with busy on-calls in radiology where, you have to prioritise which patients to image based on clinical need ensure the best possible clinical outcomes."

3.3.8 Leadership

Question
What makes a good leader?

Alternative questions
- Are you a good leader?
- What makes a good manager?
- What is this difference between leadership and management?

What the interviewers are looking for

Evidence that you have shown leadership that you can make decisions and organise and motivate other team members.

How to answer

There are many definitions of leadership, but in the context of healthcare, leadership is ultimately about driving a group to change and helping to develop others with the view to improving patient care. In order to do this, good leaders exhibit a wide range of skills, from communication to making decisions to listening to others and being supportive.

The interviewers are of course aware that you may be a FY2 Doctor and are unlikely to be a hospital Chief Executive, but that doesn't mean that you can't find everyday examples of leadership. Think about an audit you have done where you identified a problem and changed practice for the better or a busy or challenging on-call where you used leadership skills to improve the outcome for a patient.

A question with some degree of crossover would be about management. So that you answer the correct question (or indeed if you are asked about the difference between leadership and management), make sure you can define both. Management is about overseeing a group to ensure that predefined standards or values are met.

It helps to consider the difference with an example. Hospital leaders introduced a policy overnight that all NG tube placement chest radiographs had to be reported by a radiologist before they could be used, but did not involve the radiology department at all in this decision. This could be described as good leadership because people are trying to change the status quo with the aim of improving patient outcomes by reducing the risk of a never event. It is however poor management, because by not involving people crucial to this policy (the radiologists) you have not ensured that this is at all feasible based on the resources of a department that may already be very stretched.

Approach

If asked what makes a good leader you must still produce a personalised answer, citing examples of your own work. It is important to have leadership role models and you should learn as much from them as possible. However, unless specifically asked, you won't get the job if you just talk about leadership skills that other people have shown. Use your own examples.

Example

"Leadership is about encouraging a group to change and develop to try to improve patient care. A good leader needs numerous qualities and I believe I have already demonstrated several of these during my career to date. Firstly, a good leader needs to be innovative and challenge the status quo, because otherwise healthcare will stagnate. I have completed several audits that have addressed problems I have personally encountered during my clinical years. For example, as a FY1 doctor I noticed that the surgical team were not happy with the quality of reports for patients they had referred to the radiology department for abdominal ultrasound to investigate right upper quadrant pain. I lead an audit of these reports and negotiated meetings with the radiologists and sonographers about how we could improve the reports to aim to improve patient care. The re-audit has demonstrated over 90% of reports now comment on the defined standards. Good leaders are also excellent communicators. During busy on-calls on my FY2 surgical job, I ensure I am in regular contact with the FY1 on the ward and the registrar and consultant who are often in theatre. By doing this, the FY1 feels supported and the seniors are aware of any new referrals. My multisource feedback often describes

how my excellent communication skills help the team I am working in to function efficiently. Finally, good leaders are decisive. Good decisions are based on reviewing the evidence in front of you to ensure you make a sound decision. During my recent Academic Foundation placement, I conducted a systematic review on the use of deep venous stenting in obstructive chronic venous disease. By summating and critically reviewing the evidence available, I could make an informed decision about when the treatment should be considered. I published the project and it was selected as the editors pick in a renowned vascular surgery journal."

TOP TIP

 Leadership. If you are struggling think about the best leader that you know in or out of work. What characteristics do they possess that makes others listen and follow them?

3.3.9 Conflict resolution

Question
How would you resolve a conflict at work?

Alternative questions
- Give an example of a conflict you were involved in at work.
- Have you been involved in any complaints made by patients?

What the interviewers are looking for

That you can demonstrate effective communication, leadership and problem solving skills in resolving work related conflicts.

How to answer

Use a specific example of a time you resolved a conflict at work, no matter how big or small. This may be related to an issue between colleagues or it could reflect a complaint made by a patient. It is important to mention whether there is any threat to patient safety as a result of the conflict and if there is then this must be addressed first. You should then go on to describe how you gathered information, supported your colleagues and acted with empathy, before coming up with practical solutions and escalated to seniors where appropriate.

Approach

Use the STAR approach to demonstrate your conflict resolutions skills with a specific example.

Example

"During my busy cardiology FY2 job, whilst on-call in A&E, I had a bleep from one of the two ward based FY1s complaining to me that the other FY1 was not pulling their weight on the ward and was not currently answering their phone or bleep.

In order to help resolve this issue I first wanted to ensure that patient safety was not being compromised, by immediately visiting the ward and asking the FY1 and the ward nurses whether they had any concerns for patient safety. Fortunately they had no imminent concerns and the patients seemed stable, but understandably the FY1 felt under a lot of pressure with the extra workload. I needed to find out more information, but I was also concerned about the wellbeing of the other FY1 who had otherwise seemed diligent and hardworking. I therefore escalated the issue to my registrar who kindly started enquiring about the safety and whereabouts of the unaccounted FY1 with the postgraduate centre and their educational supervisor while I sat down with the other FY1 on the ward. The FY1 was concerned that it was a very busy job and they would not be able to do the job of two people for much longer. I explained that I understood their concerns and congratulated them on speaking up. My registrar discovered that the other FY1 was in the hospital, but was talking to the postgraduate manager due to some personal issues that they needed some time off to resolve. In order to support our colleagues, I suggested that I stayed on the ward and another FY2 from a less busy firm helped out with the on call. The trust was able to find a locum for the next couple of weeks, before our colleague could return. As a result, the team was stronger as both of the FY1s felt valued by their colleagues. I learnt the importance of investigating thoroughly before jumping to conclusions when resolving conflicts and I was delighted to receive excellent feedback from my supervisor with how I handled the situation."

3.3.10 Probity

Question
Tell us about a mistake you have made at work.

Alternative questions
- Show us evidence of reflection in your portfolio and explain how this has changed your practice.

What the interviewers are looking for

The interviewers want to know that you recognise your own mistakes, act quickly to rectify them, involve appropriate help and reflect on them and change for the better as a result. This is a chance for you to use a personal example to demonstrate several of the characteristics from the person specification such as integrity, taking 'responsibility for (your) own actions' and showing 'evidence of self-reflective practice'.

How to answer

You could choose a clinical or non-clinical example. A non-clinical example might be something like an error in a project you did which you then presented to your hospital before realising. The interviewers may ask you for a clinical error, but it is unlikely they would ask you for a non-clinical one specifically. Along with the fact that there is a great deal that you and others can learn from a personal clinical error, we would advise you to have a clinical example to hand.

You want to choose a real example where you genuinely did learn a lot. Be careful not to choose something that makes you sound overly incompetent. A good example could be a near miss or something causing mild harm to a patient, but the marks are scored for showing you have the awareness to recognise it, that you promptly dealt with it and that you (and ideally others as well) learnt from it. Remember to say you filled in an incident form if it is a clinical mistake.

Approach

Use the STAR approach as you are asked for a specific example:

- **Situation** – Briefly set the scene with minimal clinical information. Explain what the mistake was and what impact it had.
- **Task** – Less important here as it is obvious you had to sort out your mistake.
- **Action** – Immediate patient safety must be the most important thing initially. Mention that you asked appropriate people for help and that you started any immediate treatment or monitoring needed. Mention how, when appropriate, you explained the mistake to the patient and their relatives.
- **Result/reflection** – This is less about the result of the mistake, but more about what you learnt, with evidence of reflection and how you ensured others also learnt from the mistake e.g. discussed it at a departmental meeting.

Example

"At the start of my FY2 general surgery placement I was asked to review a patient on-call who the ward had been informed had a very low potassium blood result. I took the patient's surname and bed number over the phone. On reviewing them, I couldn't find an explanation as to why the potassium would be so low, so I ran a venous blood gas to double check the result before acting on it. This result was normal and I then realised there were two patients with the same surname and I was reviewing the wrong patient at the other end of the ward. Fortunately I was able to manage the patient who really did have a dangerously low potassium without further delay and no harm came to them.

Portfolio: 3.3.10 Probity

On realising my mistake I placed patient safety first, by immediately asking the correct patient to be placed on cardiac monitoring, whilst I promptly reviewed them. I involved my seniors by asking my registrar for help as we followed the trust guidelines on potassium correction and involved the medical team. My mistake had affected two patients and with the support of my registrar I offered an apology to the patient I had done an unnecessary blood test on and to the patient with the low potassium who I had been delayed in reviewing. Both patients were very understanding and appreciated the apology. I ensured this was all clearly documented; I handed over the specifics to the night doctor, including a plan for repeat bloods, and completed an incident form for this near miss error. Once the dust had settled, I created a reflection in my portfolio, which I can show you here, and went through this with my supervisor. I learnt just how important patient identification is and now ensure I take three pieces of identifiable information before every interaction with a patient. I also learnt the importance of placing immediate patient safety first after a clinical error occurs, but once this has been considered, I now understand that offering an explanation of the mistake and an apology can go a long way. Together with my supervisor, we helped create an electronic alert system on our computers that gives a specific message to all users when two patients with the same name are on the ward, to try and minimise the risk of a similar event happening again. Having attended a learning from discrepancy meeting during my taster week, I appreciate there is an ethos of learning from errors in radiology and tools like these are vital in order to improve our clinical practice."

4 COMMITMENT TO SPECIALTY

4.1 What are the greatest challenges facing radiology? 90
4.2 What do you think the future of radiology is? . 91
4.3 How will 7-day working affect radiology? . . . 92
4.4 How do radiologists learn from their mistakes? 93
4.5 What are the different subspecialties within radiology? 94
4.6 Tell us about radiology training 95
4.7 What is your preferred type of training scheme? 97
4.8 What is the role of the consultant radiologist? . 98
4.9 What can you bring to radiology? 99
4.10 What will you miss as a radiologist? 100
4.11 What is PACS? 101
4.12 What do you think of skills mix? 102
4.13 What are the harmful effects of ionising radiation? 103
4.14 What do you know about ionising radiation legislation in the UK? 104
4.15 What do you think of outsourcing? 105

4.1 What are the greatest challenges facing radiology?

Alternative questions

- What threats are there to radiology?
- What are your worries for the future of radiology?

How to answer

There are a number of perceived challenges or threats facing radiology which include:

- Outsourcing: external reporting of images by private companies may undercut UK radiologists, as work can be done for cheaper elsewhere.
- Skills mix: more expansive roles of radiographers may lead to less work for radiologists in the future.
- Turf wars: areas of imaging such as vascular intervention may be taken away by other hospital specialties, leaving less work for radiologists.

It is important not to sound too negative. These are challenges, and by their nature can be overcome by the hard work and creativity of future radiologists. Outsourcing and teleradiology have allowed radiologists to view images anywhere in the world, and could therefore facilitate more flexible working patterns and off-site supervision of trainees. Routine investigations could be outsourced, allowing in-house radiologists to concentrate on specialist investigations and MDT discussions. Reporting of images by radiographers could save departments money, allowing it to be channelled into other areas such as extra staff and equipment. The threat of losing work to other hospital specialties should encourage radiologists to add value to the imaging investigations they perform. Adding value can come in the form of recommending further tests or being available to discuss findings with the referring team. A good overview of the current problems faced by the specialty is contained within the RCR workforce census, the latest version of which is available online. We recommend this as essential reading prior to interview.

COMMITMENT

4.2 What do you think the future of radiology is?

Alternative questions

- Where do you see radiology going in the next 10/15/25 years?
- What are the latest innovations in radiology?

How to answer

This is a broad topic as the future of radiology in the UK remains linked to the fate of the NHS as well as to various technological developments.

Short term

As the growth in the number of imaging investigations being carried out exceeds that of the radiology workforce, radiologists will be doing more work than ever before. According to the latest RCR census, between 2012 – 15, the number of CT and MRI scans being carried out grew by 29% and 26% respectively. However, the UK currently has seven radiologists per 100,000 of the population, the third lowest of 31 European countries. At the same time, patients and their scans are becoming more complex and so each case will take more time to report. Radiology services will therefore have to become more efficient to cope with the added demands and keep up with the workload. This will likely involve more of what we have been seeing over the last few years: namely greater reliance on outsourcing and training radiographers to report their own imaging investigations.

Medium to long term

Regardless of the situation within the NHS, technological advancements will continue to drive radiology into the future. Current modalities such as CT and MRI will improve with better spatial and temporal resolution. Scanners that are currently being used solely for research purposes (e.g. 7 Tesla MRI) will move into the clinical domain. There will be further reductions in ionising radiation dose for modalities such as CT. There are likely to be further developments in functional imaging techniques such as PET-CT and PET-MRI. It would be useful to have one or two of these topics in mind prior to interview. Good resources include the two principle UK radiology journals: Radiology and the British Journal of Radiology as well as conference proceedings such as the Radiological Society of North America (RSNA). Attending a radiology conference will demonstrate your commitment to the specialty and give you useful interview fodder regarding the latest developments within the field.

4.3 How will 7-day working affect radiology?

Alternative questions

- Should there be 7-day working in radiology?
- What are the challenges of providing a 24/7 diagnostic radiology service?

How to answer

Radiology is no longer confined to 'office hours', and there is growing pressure for departments to provide services at all times. The key document to read is entitled 'Standards for providing a seven-day acute care diagnostic radiology service' (RCR, 2015) and is available online. In summary:

- Acutely ill patients require access to diagnostic radiology services at all times
- Safe radiological staffing is required to deliver satisfactory patient outcomes
- A 7-day radiology service should be provided as part of a comprehensive 7-day service by all clinical teams rather than in isolation

In terms of answering this question, few radiologists would disagree that providing a safe and effective on-call service for sick patients is important to ensuring good outcomes. The main barriers to this are inevitably: funding, staff levels and physical resources (scanners, IT systems etc.). As a trainee you will be largely responsible for ensuring that your rota is safe and takes into account the European Working Time Directive (EWTD). A slightly more contentious topic is 7-day working and the provision of non-urgent imaging on weekends. This has become a popular topic within radiology and was the subject of a 2012 Department of Health report entitled 'Implementing 7 Day working in Imaging Departments: Good Practice Guidance'. Arguments for providing a 7-day service include: more efficient use of scanners, benefitting patient choice by carrying out routine scans on weekends and reducing waiting times. However, it goes without saying that extending the 5-day week to 7 days will require more investment in staff and infrastructure. More radiologists will be required to cover rotas, and there is a worry that radiologists providing a weekend service will no longer be available during the week to provide specialist opinions. It is also the case that other clinical teams will have to adopt 7-day working in order for radiology results to be actioned in a timely manner. After all, it is no use issuing a time-critical report on a Saturday if the referring team will not read it until Monday.

4.4 How do radiologists learn from their mistakes?

Alternative questions

- What do you know about discrepancy meetings?
- What is the role of incident reporting within radiology?

How to answer

Radiologists are bound to make errors during their careers, and systems should be in place to ensure that mistakes are accounted for and lessons learnt. The system favoured by the RCR is the learning from discrepancy meeting (LDM). The term 'discrepancy' is often used because it takes into account all types of reporting error, whether radiologist-related or not. A discrepancy occurs when on retrospective review or subsequent information about patient outcome leads to an opinion different from that expressed in the original report.

LDMs are departmental meetings in which reporting discrepancies are discussed with an aim of facilitating shared learning and improving the quality of future reporting. An important part of the structure is that cases are anonymised. LDMs should occur at least every two months and attendance is recorded. It would be useful to attend an LDM in your hospital prior to the interview to get an idea of how they run. The important points to remember are the emphasis on shared learning and the maintenance of anonymity. This is explained in more detail in an RCR document entitled 'Standards for Learning from Discrepancies meetings' (2014) which is available online. As a radiologist involved in a discrepancy, you have a duty of candour to be honest and volunteer all relevant information. Important point to remember are as follows:

- The clinical team in charge of the patient need to be aware of the discrepancy
- The clinical significance and impact to the patient needs to be considered
- An incident report should be considered

An incident report should be submitted when the discrepancy is considered to be of clinical significance and this would come to light during discussion between radiology and the clinical team.

4.5 What are the different subspecialties within radiology?

Alternative questions

- What subspecialty would you like to work in?
- What are the pros and cons of subspecialisation within radiology?

How to answer

This is a bit of a trick question as technically the only recognised 'subspecialty' within radiology is interventional radiology. However, the RCR curriculum encourages trainees to pursue special areas of interest during the last two years of training. These include:

- Head and neck
- Neuroradiology
- Musculoskeletal
- Gastrointestinal/genitourinary
- Chest
- Breast
- Paediatrics

When answering, it is important to remember that those interviewing you will have a variety of special areas of interest. Balance is therefore key. If, for instance, you have lots of experience within paediatrics, you may wish to express an interest in paediatric radiology. As a core radiology trainee, this could be pursued by attending meetings and reporting sessions with a paediatric radiologist. Having one or more special areas of interest is encouraged by the RCR curriculum and is important in allowing radiologists to keep up-to-date with their specialist clinician colleagues. The main drawback of developing a special interest is a perceived loss of general radiology knowledge and skills. It is very common for applicants to express an interest in interventional radiology without mentioning the need to develop good diagnostic skills first. Nobody, least of all the interviewer, will be impressed by a candidate who wants to be skilled in a particular area to the detriment of core competencies.

4.6 Tell us about radiology training

Alternative questions

- Describe a typical day of a radiology registrar
- Is radiology training easy?
- What do you know about assessments for trainees?

How to answer

You will be expected to know that radiology training is a 5-year 'run-through' programme, with an additional 6th year for those wanting to pursue interventional radiology. Training is structured according to the RCR curriculum into core training (ST1-3) and advanced training (ST4-5). Typical expectations at each level of training are as follows:

ST1:
Modality-based blocks such as ultrasound, CT and fluoroscopy
The First FRCR exam

ST2-3:
Special interest blocks such as paediatrics, chest and neuroradiology
The Final FRCR exam (Part A)
Starting on-calls

ST4-5:
Developing one or more special areas of interest
The Final FRCR exam (Part B)
Applying for consultant/fellowship posts

It is absolutely essential that you have some knowledge of the RCR curriculum which is available online. In the 2017 interviews, candidates were questioned specifically about the assessment structure for trainees. The purpose of assessment is to enhance learning and identify areas for development. It also ensures that trainees are meeting the curriculum standards as well as those set out by the GMC. Essentially, your progress through various attachments is documented through workplace-based assessments (WpBAs) and appraisals recorded in ePortfolio and reviewed annually at the ARCP. WpBAs are a type of formative assessment and comprise:

- Mini Image Interpretation Exercise (mini-IPX) – minimum of six per year
- Radiology Direct Observation of Procedural Skills (RAD-DOPS) – minimum of six per year
- Audit assessment – minimum of one per year
- Teaching observation – minimum of two per year
- Multisource feedback (MSF) – minimum of one per year

4.6 Tell Us About Radiology Training

- MDT assessment – minimum of two per year (after ST3)

Summative assessment is provided in the form of the FRCR exams. These exams accompany each level of training and consist of two parts: the First FRCR and the Final FRCR. Knowledge of the exam structure will be expected at interview and you should make efforts to discuss their impact with current radiology trainees.

4.7 What is your preferred type of training scheme?

Alternative questions

- Describe the different styles of radiology training
- What do you think of radiology academies?

How to answer

Broadly speaking, there are two types of training scheme: apprenticeship-style schemes and radiology academies. It is likely that most applicants will have undertaken a taster week within a radiology department and so will be familiar with the more traditional apprenticeship-style of learning. You may be less familiar with the radiology academies. Important points are as follows:

- There are currently three academies: Norwich, Leeds and Peninsula
- The notion of academies is to increase radiology training numbers in response to a 2002 RCR publication entitled 'Clinical radiology: A workforce in Crisis'
- Academies are physically separate from the main radiology department
- Time is divided between the educational environment and the clinical environment
- There is an emphasis on e-learning using R-ITI, lectures and clinical skills simulations

Both styles of training have their advantages and disadvantages and it is up to the applicant to decide which is best suited to them. It is worth considering that the academy style of training is currently mandated by the RCR and those interviewing you may practice in such a scheme. It would therefore be wise to have some knowledge of how the academies work and provide a balanced opinion on the positives and negatives of training in one.

Advantages of academy training include:
- Exposure to numerous 'cold' cases which are hand-picked to demonstrate specific pathologies
- Freedom to make mistakes at an early stage of training
- Training can be standardised across schemes and set to match the RCR curriculum

Disadvantages include:
- A lack of early exposure to time-pressured or 'hot' reporting
- Difficulty delivering hands-on training such as intervention or ultrasound (although simulators are becoming available)
- Less time spent working with senior colleagues and other members of the department e.g. radiographers

4.8 What is the role of the consultant radiologist?

Alternative questions

- Describe a day in the life of a consultant radiologist
- What is the role of the radiologist at the MDTM?

How to answer

Interviewers will expect you to understand that the role of the consultant radiologist involves more than just reporting scans. The best way to answer this question involves referring to your taster week and thinking back to your experiences with consultant radiologists. It may be useful to divide the role of the consultant radiologist using the CAMP structure:

Clinical:
Reporting scans
Carrying out interventional work
Leading MDTMs

Academic:
Teaching registrars and medical students
Research activities
Audit

Management:
Organising rotas
Responsibility for departmental budgets
Appointing new members of staff

Personal:
Mentoring and supervision roles

Each consultant radiologist has a predetermined job plan which is in accordance with the NHS consultant contract. For a full-time consultant, the 40-hour week is divided into 10 planned activities (PAs). A typical balance is 7.5 PAs for direct clinical care (reporting, preparing for and attending MDTMs, supervising trainees) and 2.5 PAs for supporting professional activities (audit, research, clinical governance). Direct clinical care also includes on-call duties which will vary between departments. You will not really be expected to know this much detail at interview, but it will help you understand why most consultant radiologists seem so busy all the time!

4.9 What can you bring to radiology?

Alternative questions

- How has your experience so far prepared you for radiology?
- What have you done so far that shows you can do well in radiology?

How to answer

This question could just as similarly be asked in the portfolio station and tests the attributes that you think will make you a good radiologist. Whichever personal attribute you select should related to a specific part of the person specification and referenced against examples in your CV. Think about your individual background and how it makes you stand out against other candidates. You do not need to include more than one clinical and one extra-curricular achievement. Examples include:

Qualifications:
Full MRCP/MRCS/MRCPCH demonstrating strong performances in postgraduate exams

Clinical experience:
A depth of clinical experience may be more relevant if applying to radiology from a more senior role

Clinical skills:
A strong procedural logbook demonstrating interest in interventional procedures

Academic skills:
Strong research or audit background focusing on patient safety and clinical improvement
Teaching course or qualification

Personal skills:
Experience in NHS management
Effective leadership outside of medicine

4.10 What will you miss as a radiologist?

Alternative questions

- How is radiology different from your current specialty?

How to answer

This is a commonly asked question and will give the interviewers an impression of how hard you have actually thought about pursuing a career in radiology. It is important to recognise that however fantastic radiology is, there are certain aspects of the job you are bound to find difficult. It is always best to discuss your fears with practicing radiologists and let the interviewers know you have done so. Although it is very much down to opinion, some of the following points are worth considering:

- Radiologists have reduced patient contact compared to most other specialties
- Radiology is predominantly a diagnostic specialty (although there is now growing scope to provide treatments)
- Radiologists often don't receive the credit (we feel they deserve!) for the diagnoses they make
- It can be difficult for radiologists to see the impact of the decisions they make aside from reporting follow-up scans

Whatever answer you give, it is always best to finish on a positive note. For instance, if you state that patient contact is limited in radiology you could go on to state that the contact is particularly meaningful because you are providing an important diagnosis and changing the direction of treatment for that patient.

4.11 What do you think of skills mix?

Alternative questions

- What are the pros and cons of extended roles for radiographers?
- What do you think of the standard of reports by radiographers?

How to answer

This is something you should be familiar with from spending time in a radiology department and meeting radiographers who have adopted reporting roles. Essentially, skills mix is viewed positively by the RCR and you should be able to emphasise the benefits to radiologists, patients and to the department as a whole. Radiographers are highly trained and undergo postgraduate education and accreditation in order to achieve advanced or consultant practitioner level. Contrary to what some radiologists may believe, they are responsible and accountable for their own reports. Advantages of skills mix include:

- Radiologist workload is reduced, especially in high-volume areas such as A&E plain films
- It is more cost-effective for radiology departments to employ radiographers to report rather than outsource to private reporting companies
- Radiographers gain additional responsibility and may value the opportunity for extra career-progression

There are a number of disadvantages to radiographer-issued reports which may include the need for consultants to review them, leading to the phenomenon of 'double reporting'. This may be beneficial in areas such as mammography where two reports are actually required. As a prospective radiology trainee, you may also want to protect your training opportunities by keeping high volume work such as A&E plain films and ultrasound. Essentially, it is about providing a balance in dividing the reporting caseload between the professions. The important document to read on the topic is entitled 'Team working in clinical imaging' (2012) and was written by the RCR in conjunction with the Society and College of Radiographers. '

4.12 What is PACS?

Alternative questions

- How do radiologists view and report images?
- What is RIS?

How to answer

PACS stands for Picture Archiving and Communication Systems and is an IT system used by radiologists to transfer, display and manipulate digital images. Images are displayed in a standardised digital imaging and communication in medicine (DICOM) format.

RIS stands for Radiology Information Systems and is an IT system used to generate radiology reports which are linked to PACS images. It contains patient information and is used to manage and schedule appointments in the radiology department. RIS is an important administrative tool and is linked to PACS to provide seamless transfer of information.

4.13 What are the harmful effects of ionising radiation?

Alternative questions

- What are the different types of radiation damage?
- How would you counsel a patient regarding the risks of ionising radiation?

How to answer

As an applicant to clinical radiology, you are possibly months away from authorising high dose imaging investigations which have the potential to cause harm to patients. Those that cause the most harm involve ionising radiation – a form of electromagnetic radiation that causes structural damage to DNA. This damage occurs either directly through the breaking of molecular bonds or indirectly through free radical production and subsequent cell membrane damage. The form of ionising radiation you will become most familiar with will be x-rays (although neutrons, alpha and beta particles are also types of ionising radiation). The effects of ionising radiation are divided into two categories:

Deterministic effects:
- Appear above a given threshold
- The severity of the effect increases with dose
- Effects occur within a short timeframe after exposure
- Examples include: skin erythema, hair loss, cataracts

Stochastic effects:
- No threshold
- The probability of the effect occurring increases with dose
- Effects may occur after a long time-lag
- Examples include: cancer, genetic mutations

Effective doses of ionising radiation are measured in Sieverts (Sv). This takes into account the radiation energy absorbed, the type of radiation, and the radiosensitivity of the irradiated tissues. High dose investigations include CT scans of the chest and abdomen and require more stringent vetting by radiologists. At diagnostic levels, doses are generally safe and patients should be reassured that benefits normally outweigh the risks. More care should be taken with younger patients and those returning for multiple scans (e.g. Crohn's patients).

4.14 What do you know about ionising radiation legislation in the UK?

Alternative questions

- What is IRMER?
- What is IRR 99?

How to answer

There are two important pieces of legislation you should be aware of prior to interview: The Ionising Radiation (Medical Exposure) Regulations 2000 (IRMER) and the Ionising Radiation Regulations 1999 (IRR 99). IRMER relates to the protection of patients, whilst IRR 99 relates largely to the protection of staff and members of the public. According to IRMER, there are four 'duty holders' who hold responsibility for protecting patients from the harmful effects of radiation. These are:

- The employer: normally an NHS trust
- The referrer: a registered healthcare professional who is able to refer a patient for a medical exposure (e.g. a GP)
- The practitioner: a registered healthcare professional whose primary responsibility is justification and authorisation of the medical exposure (normally a radiologist)
- The operator: a person who undertakes the practical aspects of the medical exposure (e.g. a radiographer)

Under IRMER, the employer has overall responsibility for radiation protection. The duty of the referrer is to provide adequate clinical information to the practitioner. The duty of the practitioner is to use this information to justify a medical exposure, taking into account the risks and benefits to the patient. Once a decision has been made, the imaging test should be optimised to provide the lowest dose possible to provide an accurate diagnosis. The overriding principle of optimisation is to keep dose as low as reasonably practicable (ALARP). The operator then carries out the medical exposure and further ensures that dose is optimised.

IRR 99 is a set of legislation made under the Health and Safety and Work Act 1974 and is designed to protect staff and members of the public from the harmful effects of radiation. It is enforced by the Health and Safety Executive (HSE). Like IRMER, it sets out a number of important roles:

- Radiation protection advisor (RPA): a medical physics expert employed by the trust who advises on all aspects of radiation protection
- Radiation protection supervisor (RPS): usually a senior radiographer involved in day-to-day management of radiation protection

IRR 99 sets out a number of effective and equivalent dose limits for workers and members of the public. Any worker who is likely to exceed a specified dose limit is known as a classified worker and is subject to annual medical checks. Areas within the radiology department may also be designated into controlled areas and supervised areas according to the dose limits which are likely to be exceeded.

4.15 What do you think of outsourcing?

Alternative questions

- What is teleradiology?
- Should radiologists be allowed to work from home?

How to answer

Teleradiology and outsourcing have been made possible by advances in technology which have allowed radiologists to view images in remote locations. The need for outsourcing has been exacerbated by significant gaps in the consultant radiologist workforce and the year-on-year increase in the volume of imaging being carried out. Essentially, you should aim to convey a balanced and well-informed opinion on outsourcing. The radiologist interviewing you may have a fixed view on outsourcing and it would be best to answer with caution. Reasons for outsourcing include:

- Out-of-hours and emergency scans can be reported in a timely fashion in hospitals without a full on-call rota
- On-call reporting volumes can be reduced, allowing radiologists to provide a full in-hours service
- Specific investigations (e.g. plain films) can be outsourced, allowing in-house radiologists to concentrate on their own areas of expertise

Problems with outsourcing include: cost, reduced efficiency and the removal of valuable training opportunities from registrars. You may have witnessed during your taster week that a high volume of interesting learning cases are scanned overnight and over the weekend. A possible solution to expensive outsourcing (and one favoured by the RCR) is to use radiology networks. A Network Teleradiology Platform (NTP) would involve several trusts sharing reporting capacity. This could involve out-of-hours reporting or more specialist areas such as head and neck or paediatric radiology being taken on by a large trust in order to support smaller trusts. This would save a considerable amount of money when compared to paying a private teleradiology provider. This is summarised in a 2016 RCR document entitled 'Who shares wins: efficient, collaborative radiology solutions'.

5 THE OLD INTERVIEW STATIONS

5.1 Report critique **107**

5.2 Ethical scenarios **115**
   5.2.1 Difficult procedure. 115
   5.2.2 Drunk colleague 117
   5.2.3 Scanning in pregnancy 119
   5.2.4 Confidentiality 121
   5.2.5 Radiation protection incident 124
   5.2.6 Contrast reaction 126
   5.2.7 Jehovah's Witness 128
   5.2.8 Inappropriate referral 130

5.1 Report Critique

Critiquing a report is a difficult task and even during specialty training there is little formal teaching on what exactly makes a good report. As with many things, the experience of practicing and reading other reports helps develop one's own reporting skills and personal style. There are however some basic structures and concepts that should be considered. In the run up to the interview, we would advise you to reflect on the radiology reports you read during your daily working practice and practice critiquing them using our suggested framework.

A framework: What makes a good radiology report?

The RCR state that, "the purpose of the report is to provide a timely answer to the clinical questions posed, together with an assessment of the whole image for relevant and/or unexpected findings." They also describe the need for clarity and for reports to be tailored to the referrer's level of familiarity. With the RCR recommendations in mind, our framework for the report critique suggests you should focus your analysis in the areas described below. As for many tasks asking you to analyse something, we believe it makes sense to consider the strengths and weaknesses of the report with suggestions for improvement.

Report structure

Using a clear structure provides the reporter with a framework for producing a succinct report that answers the clinical questions and will be appreciated by the referrer. Clearly not all radiological studies require a detailed structured report. For example, a finger radiograph may just require a binary answer for the presence or absence of a bony injury. More complex studies however will likely benefit from a clear, structured report.

A report structure such as the one recommended in the American College of Radiology (ACR) Residents Guide is widely seen in daily practice and is explored in more detail below.

1) Clinical history
By acknowledging and documenting the provided clinical history and/or a clinical question(s), the reporting radiologist makes it clear to the referrer that they are interpreting the radiological findings in light of the clinical history.

2) Technique
A comment on technique is not always required, for example it may be less relevant for an outpatient GP study. At other times, where there is a close daily interaction between the radiologists and clinicians, stating whether a contrast agent has been given, what phases were acquired or what MRI sequences were used may help provide the referrer with reassurance that the correct study was done to answer their question.

3) Comparison

Previous studies often provide vital information to the reporting radiologist. Reports should list the imaging studies that the current study has been compared to.

4) Findings

The radiological findings should include a clear, relevant description of any abnormalities. It is logical to mention the most important findings at the start of the report. The description itself should include things like the location, size, shape and radiological characteristics. One common mistake in the findings section is that the findings are also immediately interpreted leading to an illogical and verbose report that may repeat itself. Often, the findings are less certain and it is important to be aware of the difference between a description of findings and an interpretation or diagnosis. For example, "smooth interlobular septal thickening with ground-glass shadowing in a perihilar distribution" is a descriptive term that may have several causes. Immediately including a wide differential diagnosis in the findings section would lead to a long, confusing report, that could be improved by leaving this until the 'impression' section (see below) where the findings are interpreted in light of the clinical information.

If measurements of any findings are included it is important that they are relevant. Measurements are likely to be relevant for an oncologist assessing tumour response to therapy, yet less relevant for a GP for whom the overall picture is more important. The importance of brevity and relevance for a report cannot be overstated. Where negative or incidental findings are included, it is important that they are relevant to the posed clinical question.

5) Impression

Arguably the most important section and this may be the only section that the clinician will read. An 'impression' or 'conclusion' may not always be required if the report in itself is particularly short, but it is likely that for the purpose of an interview you would be given a longer report, where an 'impression' section could potentially be helpful.

Fundamentally, the 'impression' should attempt to answer the clinical question. If the study is normal, a reference should still be made to the clinical question, rather than just stating that the examination is normal. This ensures the referrer is aware the radiologist understood the question they wanted answering and did not miss the point. Where it is not possible to give a definitive answer or make a specific diagnosis, the degree of certainty of the findings should be qualified and a relevant differential diagnosis could be given. It is not helpful to give an endless list of differentials as this may make the referrer feel the radiologist is particularly uncertain about the findings.

The ACR recommend a final section of 'communication'. This is often included in or beneath the 'impression' section.

Report style and content – relevance, brevity and hedging

Naturally, radiologists' reporting styles will vary amongst individuals. However, there are three key points to consider when assessing the reporting style and content during the preparation station:

1) Relevance
This is of particular importance to the 'findings' section of a structured report and was touched upon in our analysis. When describing findings and listing points in the 'impression' section it makes sense to list them in order of importance to draw the clinician's attention to them. Listing endless negatives or normal variants should be avoided.

2) Brevity
This is relevant to the whole report and brevity should generally be strived for to produce a more readable report. There are times when longer descriptions of findings may be required, for example where there is diagnostic uncertainty, a broad description helps to "show your working" as to whether you think the finding is important and how urgently something should be done about it.

3) Hedging
Hedging is something you have probably come across in radiology reports and is when a radiologist uses ambiguous language to avoid being wrong. Whilst this may leave the radiologist feeling reassured that they cannot be accountable for what they have said, it provides a less helpful report for the clinician and ultimately the patient. An example would be, "no suspicious lung nodules are seen." The use of the word "suspicious" may imply some non-suspicious nodules that may still need something doing about them. It is better to say "no nodules" or if there are other nodules that are not worrying, to describe them and then dismiss them. Also, by saying that no nodules are "seen" implies there are nodules, but you can't see them on the scan or that you have just missed them.

It is not wrong to include some hedging phrases, but an overly hedged report will come across as rather unconvincing. That is not to say one should be overly bold with reports in a black and white manner either. A balance between the two approaches would be to try and avoid hedged terms where possible, but where there is diagnostic uncertainty to state this.

Medico-legal document

Finally it must be remembered that the radiology report is a legal document, exactly the like documentation on the wards and in theatres and this has several implications. The RCR have produced clear guidelines for hospitals in terms of the standards for the communication of radiology reports based on a National Patient Safety Agency report. The guidelines list several standards and three are particularly relevant to radiologists:

The Old Interview Stations: 5.1 Report Critique

1) "Radiologists should ensure that the reports are timely, clear and precise, and the urgency for action is clearly documented within the content of the report"

This encompasses much of what has been described above in terms of produces a concise, readable report. It is also important to consider errors in the report, particularly in the era of reporting with voice recognition software. Proofreading reports is vital to avoid errors that may otherwise be acted on by clinicians. Another important point is abbreviations – use only the most conventional ones as less common ones can lead to confusion at best or at worst, harm for the patient if misinterpreted.

2) "Radiologists should clearly document advice on further management or action, where appropriate"

Particularly with critical findings that must be acted on immediately.

3) "Radiologists should inform verbally (by telephone) the appropriate referring clinician/team of an unexpected acute life- or limb-threatening finding which requires emergency clinical action. He/she should document that this was done, (when and to who) within the radiology report or via an addendum"

Hospitals are expected to have alert systems to highlight unexpected or important findings such as cancer and these are appropriate for outpatient settings. Whilst it is the legal responsibility of the clinicians to read and act on radiology reports, it is best practice by the radiologist to pick up the phone and contact someone if the clinicians should know something there and then – for example an acute pulmonary embolism or an abdominal bleed. If a phone call is made, this should be documented in the report, just as you would document something with an entry into a patient's notes.

Our suggested framework for approaching the report critique is summarised in Figure 1. Below we apply the framework to two worked examples of reports of varying qualities. Read through the examples and apply the framework. We present the summary key arguments you could make at interview. When making your arguments, personalising your answer to demonstrate that you read and thought about what makes a good report is recommended as this shows you not only have an interest in radiology, but are also intent on becoming a good radiologist.

The Old Interview Stations: 5.1 Report Critique

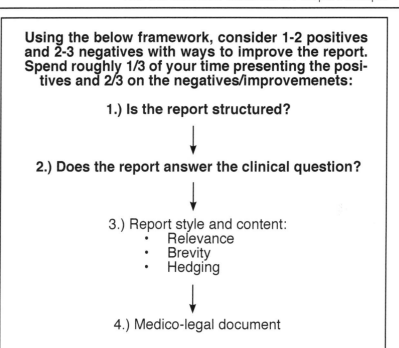

Figure 1. A suggested framework for preparing your report critique.

Report number 1

Outpatient scan requested by a GP. The patient is a 72-year-old male.

Information available to the reporting radiologist:
• Request form "11 kg weight loss, abdominal pain 6/12, ?malignancy"
• Two previous CT thorax, abdomen and pelvis scans on PACS

"CT thorax, abdomen and pelvis

There is an azygous lobe and also a left horizontal fissure. There are some possible small opacities within the right upper zone that may represent some small nodules. The significance of these is uncertain and clinical correlation is advised. The differential diagnosis includes infection, inflammation, malignancy, haemorrhage or aspiration. There are no suspicious masses. No pleural or pericardial effusions. The airway, aortic arch and great vessels are intact. The patient is not intubated. No significant axillary, supraclavicular, superior mediastinal, inferior mediastinal, hilar or retrocrural lymphadenopathy. The liver appears normal. The CBD measures 7 mm. The gallbladder, pancreas and spleen have unremarkable appearances, aside from a small splenunculus. The kidneys demonstrate no obvious hydronephrosis or masses. There is a 6 mm left adrenal nodule. The urinary bladder is underfilled, but demonstrates a generally thick wall and even accounting for the lack of distension there is there

The Old Interview Stations: 5.1 Report Critique

is thick walls abnormal. There is no bowel preparation, but there are no obvious sinister lesions of the colon. Clinical correlation advised. No significant inguinal, pelvic, retroperitoneal or mesenteric lymphadenopathy. Bone review demonstrates a well-defined lucency within the left iliac wing of uncertain significance or aetiology and this may need further investigation. There are anterior wedge compression fractures of T10 and T11 of uncertain chronicity."

Clearly there are several problems with this report and we have tried to highlight everything you could comment on. Below is a model answer for presenting a critique of the report that is based on our framework and encompasses the most important parts:

"Whilst there are some strengths of this report, there are several more weaknesses and areas for improvement.

One strength is that, given the clinical team's suspicion for a malignancy, the report does state several important negatives. For example, the absence of "pleural or pericardial effusions", an "unremarkable" appearing pancreas and the lack of significant abdominal lymphadenopathy are all **relevant** *negatives in the context of someone who may have cancer.*

However, there are several fundamental flaws. Firstly, the lack of **structure** *makes the report very difficult to read. The best reports that I have read during my clinical practice document a clear clinical history that makes you aware that the radiologist is interpreting the images in light of the clinical picture, which I find reassuring. They also give a separate section for the findings which describe what the images show, but more importantly, they give a clear conclusion or impression at the end. This report lacks this vital section and as a result there is no recommendation about what to do about the described findings. It also means that there is no clear* **answer to the clinical question**, *but just a list of findings with no clear clinical implication.*

Secondly, the report gives several examples of **hedging**. *Hedging can be defined as using vague language to remain non-committal. Whilst this may mean that the radiologist is not wrong, it is not helpful for the clinicians and I find it may decrease my trust in the report. A specific example in this report is the vague description of the "possible nodules", the wide differential and recommending clinical correlation. In terms of improvement, where there is uncertainty, I find the use of the first person in the report a nice personal touch that helps illustrate the radiologist's thinking and earmarking helpful radiological meetings for further discussion is always useful.*

Finally, much like documentation on the ward, the radiological report is an important **medico-legal document**. *As such, it should be clear and the typographical errors regarding the bladder means it is not clear whether this is significant pathology or not and the clinician may or may not act appropriately as a result of this. It is vital that reports are proof-read before authorisation.*

In summary, there are some strengths to the report in terms of the important negatives, but the lack of structure, the lack of an answer to the clinical question, the hedged descriptions and the key spelling mistake mean that there are several areas for improvement."

Report number 2

Inpatient scan requested by the acute medical team. The patient is a 63-year-old male.

Information available to the reporting radiologist:
• Request form "sudden onset pleuritic chest pain and SOB. Raised d-dimer, hypoxic ?PE"
• A chest radiograph performed the same day is available on PACS.

"CTPA

Clinical information: "Sudden onset pleuritic chest pain and SOB. Raised d-diner, hypoxic ?PE"

Technique: Pulmonary arterial phase contrast enhanced acquisition with multi-planar reformats.

Comparison: Nil previous cross-sectional studies. Chest radiograph performed the same day.

Findings: Satisfactory opacification of the pulmonary arterial tree. There is a filling defect within the left lower lobe pulmonary artery that is consistent with a PE. No other filling defects detected to suggest further PEs and no abnormal bowing of the interventricular septum and the pulmonary trunk diameter measures 25 mm.

The parenchymal lung appearances are significantly degraded by movement artefact. Accounting for this, the lung parenchyma appears grossly unremarkable, although it would be difficult to exclude small nodules. No pleural or pericardial effusions. No enlarged axillary, supraclavicular or intrathoracic lymph nodes.

Beneath the diaphragm, assessment of the imaged viscera is difficult due to the phase of contrast enhancement. Accounting for this, there is no obvious gross abnormality, but clinical correlation is advised.

On bony review, there is extensive anterior flowing osteophytosis with preserved adjacent intervertebral disc spaces consistent with DISH.

Impression:

1. Left lower lobe pulmonary artery filling defect consistent with a PE.
2. Accounting for the described technical inadequacies the remainder of the thorax appears unremarkable.

The Old Interview Stations: 5.1 Report Critique

The findings were communicated to the clinical team.

Dr Joe Bloggs
Consultant Radiologist"

This report clearly demonstrates many more good points than the previous one and we present again a model answer based on the framework.

"This report demonstrates several strengths, but there are still a couple of minor negatives with areas for improvement.

One of the strongest positives about this report is the clear **structure** *it uses. In my current clinical practice, I find structured, logically laid out reports much easier to read and I find it increases my satisfaction with the report. Specifically in this case, the documentation of the clinical history is reassuring to the referrer that the radiologist is interpreting the findings in light of the clinical information. The impression section at the end also mentions the most important points, so that even if the clinician only reads this section, then the pertinent points have been conveyed. The use of a structure makes it much easier for the report to clearly* **answer the clinical question.**

Another strength is the **relevance and brevity** *of the report. Examples of the relevance are the important negatives that it mentions after describing the PE in terms of the signs of right heart strain in the context of a PE. The report is reasonably short, which makes it digestible. This is in part due to the succinct descriptions used and the absence of a string of sentences beginning with "there is" or "there are" and the lack of irrelevant negatives.*

However, there are also a couple of key negatives. **Hedging** *refers to using vague, non-committal terms that mean the radiologist cannot be shown to be wrong, but they are not always helpful for the clinician. This report demonstrates a couple of examples, for example the use of "no obvious gross abnormality" and recommending "clinical correlation" when describing the abdomen. A CTPA is not designed to assess abdominal organs and the clinician doesn't mention the suspicion of abdominal pathology. The hedged terms may therefore confuse or worry the clinician and lead to unnecessary investigations. A phrase such as "unremarkable appearance of the imaged abdominal organs for the phase of study" may be more helpful.*

Finally, the radiology report is an important **medico-legal document** *and the Royal College of Radiologists have produced clear guidelines about when to contact the referrer and how this must be documented in the report. In this case, the radiologist does contact the referrer, but the documentation is suboptimal, as it does not describe who, how or when they contacted. Good documentation also avoids using unusual abbreviations and to my knowledge the use of "DISH" is not typical.*

In summary, this is generally a very good report, largely because it has a clear

5.2 Ethnical Scenarios

5.2.1 Difficult procedure

Scenario

You are the senior interventional radiology (IR) registrar on-call overnight. You are asked to perform an emergency coil embolisation on a patient who has been involved in an RTC. You have assisted in similar procedures before but have not performed one independently. You attempt to contact your consultant through the switchboard but receive no answer.

Questions
How would you approach this scenario?

Seek information and Patient safety: Patient safety is key here. You need to ascertain whether the patient is stable and how urgent this procedure truly is. Can the patient be optimised while you get hold of the consultant? Is there another consultant who can assist you or another senior IR registrar who is able to perform the procedure? Remember that is easy to assume you would be ok if everything were to go to plan, but should a complication occur that is beyond your competency level you have no senior cover and it could turn quickly into a dangerous situation.

Initiative: Ensure you have tried all available methods of communication. Switchboard may have multiple contact numbers and sometimes the on-call IR nurses will have alternative contact details. Check contact details on notice boards. Consider whether there is an alternative (e.g. surgery) that would achieve a similar outcome. Close communication with the clinical team here is essential.

Escalate: Contact the diagnostic radiology consultant on call for advice. If you cannot reach the IR consultant on second attempt, escalate according to local guidelines, usually to the head of department (who will likely not be on-call but will be receptive to this sort of situation), even up to medical director level.

What are the key issues?

When you are on-call you should never be expected to or pressured into performing a procedure that you are not competent, safe or comfortable to do. It is neither in the patient's best interest, nor yours, to risk it by "just having a go". This station tests your probity and your ability to recognise the limits of your own competency under pressure. Secondly, inability to communicate with non-resident on-call senior colleagues is a very realistic situation and one you might come across easily in any clinical situation so is excellent fodder for interview.

You reach the consultant eventually who states that he is over an hour and a half away, probably two hours, due to traffic.

You need to decide whether this is time that you have. If the patient is unstable could they be optimised with IV fluids and transfusion in the meantime? Again, close discussion with the clinical team is essential and it is likely a consultant-level decision would be necessary. It would be a good idea if the consultant looking after the patient and the IR consultant were to communicate directly. In the meantime, you could ensure that the patient is worked up for the procedure, consented and the IR suite prepared.

The consultant starts the procedure and you notice that he is not performing it as you have seen others do the procedure. You think this is an old-fashioned method that is not evidence-based. What do you do?

GMC Duties of a doctor state that doctors must keep professional knowledge and skills up to date in order to provide a good standard of practice and care. Do you think this consultant has done this? If you feel it is unsafe, you should sensitively address your concerns during the procedure. There may well be a good reason for the method the consultant is using, or he/she may have not considered a preferred option. If you think patient safety is truly compromised you should stop the procedure and escalate. Take care not to cause distraction, perhaps by asking at a natural pause in the procedure. The ability to speak up as a junior colleague when you notice something that may be detrimental to patient safety is very important. Much is being done within healthcare to breed the kind of environment where anyone can highlight a safety concern and this falls under the umbrella term of Clinical Human Factor management.

How can you keep your professional knowledge and skills up to date?

Continuing professional development is key to patient safety. During your training it is easy to keep knowledge and skills up to date by attending teaching, completing exams and learning from senior colleagues on a day-to-day basis. Attendance at conferences, courses and reading journals to keep abreast of latest research developments is also useful. Interviewers may ask you if there are any journals or online resources you read regularly.

Following the procedure you see the IR nurse changing the patient with the curtains around the bed open. What should you do?

GMC Duties of a doctor state that one must act immediately if patient safety, dignity or comfort is being compromised. Therefore, the first step is to simply close the curtains. Once the nurse is finished you should sensitively discuss your concerns about maintaining patient dignity directly with them.

The nurse states that he was very busy and frankly doesn't have time to faff around with the curtains. What do you do?

You could discuss the importance of patient dignity with him. If your concerns persist or you see that he continues to treat patients with a lack of respect you should escalate this to the IR department manager. This scenario highlights the difference in hierarchy between different members of the multidisciplinary team and it is worth considering prior to your interview how to escalate appropriately in a variety of situations.

Summary

This scenario touches on a variety of ethical and management points. The interviewers will want to see that you will not be pressured into performing an unsafe procedure and can appropriately communicate with the clinical team about it whilst maintaining patient safety.

TOP TIPS

- Know the limits of your competency
- Have an awareness of the expected limits of junior and senior radiology registrars

5.2.2 Drunk colleague

Scenario

Your supervising consultant arrives at the morning CT list smelling of alcohol and is clearly intoxicated. What do you do?

Questions

How would you approach this scenario?

Seek Information: Talk to the consultant to gain more information in a sensitive manner – is he intoxicated or is there some other explanation? Good communication is vital here as it is an incredibly challenging situation, especially when involving a senior colleague.

Patient safety: Whilst at first it might seem that radiology is slightly removed from patient safety, we must remember that significant patient decisions are made based on radiology reports that we provide, so any inaccuracies resulting from the consultant's intoxication may cause patient harm.

Initiative: Simply opening the discussion with the consultant may raise awareness that he/she is unfit to work and it is likely that at this stage they would go home.

Escalation: It is critical that, even if the consultant leaves, this is escalated to

The Old Interview Stations: 5.2.2 Drunk Colleague

someone senior that can deal with the longer-term consequences of this scenario. Your line manager or the department clinical director would be appropriate people to approach. If the colleague in question is the clinical director or your line manager then you must escalate to a level more senior than this, you could approach your educational supervisor for assistance in whom to contact.

Support: It is easy to forget about your colleague in this scenario but support should be considered once patient safety concerns are allayed. This incident may have career-changing consequences and appropriate support should be offered to the consultant in managing the potential underlying problems which have resulted in this incident. However, this is probably best coming from a peer rather than someone at your level.

What are the key issues?

It is key to remember that critical decisions are made based on the reports that we provide to clinicians and, as such, patient safety is always the first consideration in this type of scenario. This scenario also highlights the importance of sensitive communication and your ability to recognise and appropriately deal with problems involving senior colleagues.

The consultant brushes off your concerns when you approach him so you approach your line manager who says "Ah, this is a long-standing issue. Please keep this to yourself" and the consultant continues with the CT list. What do you do?

What are your concerns here? There is still a risk to patient safety and this is clearly an unacceptable response to your totally legitimate concerns and further escalation is necessary. You might try discussing your concerns regarding patient safety and the consultant continuing with the CT list with your line manager, escalating higher or escalating to outside the radiology department, although this would be a last resort.

You are reviewing some of the morning CT scans for your own learning. The consultant did not go home and you notice that he has signed off a CT as normal but has missed a malignancy on the scan. What do you do?

Your first concern here is confirming this discrepancy. Sensitively approach the consultant who wrote the initial report, highlight your concern and confirm whether or not you are correct. If the consultant is not available, get the scan reviewed for a second opinion by another consultant and ensure that an addendum is added. This will need to be communicated directly with the clinical team to highlight the discrepancy in the event that clinical decisions have been made based on the initial full scan report. This scenario also goes one step further than just the recognition of discrepancy in that there is potentially an implication that the consultant was not fit to be working at the time. Escalation to senior management in this case is essential.

Summary

Dealing with problems involving senior colleagues is a common scenario at interview. You should act in the patient's best interest by addressing the issue early and keeping patient safety your priority.
Discrepancy is an everyday part of life in radiology and the interviewers will want you to demonstrate your integrity in reporting your own discrepancies as well as those of others as well as your ability to communicate this to the clinical team.

5.2.3 Scanning in pregnancy

Scenario
You are the ST2 radiologist reporting CT. The radiographer informs you that after undergoing an abdominal CT scan, a 21-year-old woman says she may be pregnant. How do you proceed?

Questions
How would you approach this scenario?

Seek information: There are a number of points to clarify in this scenario and information should be gathered both from the radiographer and the patient. Most importantly, was the patient asked if there was a possibility she could be pregnant prior to the scan? Other considerations include the patient's reasons for suspecting pregnancy, the indication for the scan and the dose received by the patient. All the above should be clearly documented.

Patient safety: Assuming the patient is not acutely unwell she is not in immediate danger, however reporting of the scan should not be delayed. Symptoms such as abdominal pain may have new significance in view of the information the patient has provided.

Initiative: With the patient's consent, the referring doctor should be informed about what has happened. It will be necessary for the patient to be appropriately assessed and to have a pregnancy test.

Escalate: This is potentially a serious incident. In the first instance, you should inform the consultant radiologist supervising you and the superintendent radiographer. The radiation protection adviser (RPA) should be informed who will be responsible for calculating the fetal dose and advising the mother on the risks. The radiation protection supervisor (RPS) should also be involved to carry out an investigation into what happened. An incident form should also be completed.

Support: The patient will be counselled appropriately by the RPA on the potential risks of fetal irradiation in the context of the scan she has received. It is important to apologise if the appropriate checks were not done. Relevant information should also be sent to the referring doctor or GP so that on-going support can be provided if necessary.

What are the key issues?

This station tests your knowledge of IRMER. You should have some knowledge about the risks associated with ionising radiation in pregnancy and the precautions taken to reduce these within the radiology department. In addition, this station asks you to deal with a situation where the department may have treated a patient inappropriately so requiring you to demonstrate honesty, professionalism and strong communication skills.

The patient asks if a baby could be seen on the scan she has just had

The patient is likely to be anxious. You should view the images with the consultant radiologist supervising you. In early pregnancy, the gestational sac maybe be visible within the pelvis on ultrasound, however it would be best to assess for pregnancy with conventional investigations such as history, urinary pregnancy test and blood beta-HCG.

The patient asks what risk there could be to her baby if she is pregnant

A CT scan of the abdomen gives a typical fetal dose of 1-10 mGy; depending on gestation this can increase the chance of childhood cancers, mental retardation, gross malformation or miscarriage to varying degrees. Although you may not know these details you would be expected to escalate to the supervising consultant radiologist so that the patient can be appropriately counselled. Often the departmental medical physicist will play a role in this as well.

What is IRMER?

IRMER is legislation to protect patients from hazards associated with ionising radiation. Concerning pregnancy, it details the need to enquire about pregnancy in relevant patients. The employer should provide a procedure for this and the appropriate inspectorate notified if there is a failure to comply.

Do you know about the 10-day or 28-day rules?

In situations where the patient is unsure about their pregnancy status, some departments use a 10-day rule in which high dose scans (e.g. CT scans of the abdomen or pelvis) are done within the first 10 days of a menstrual cycle as it is unlikely the patient will be pregnant then. For other scans, a 28-day rule is used whereby the scan is carried out if the patient's period is not overdue.

The patient does not recall being asked about pregnancy prior to the scan, the radiographer however is insistent that she was, however there is no documentation of this.

This is a difficult situation as you are being given conflicting accounts of what has happened. The IRMER regulations state that the response to pregnancy enquiries should be clearly documented. This is not a situation you will be able to deal with alone therefore it is important to escalate to the superintendent radiographer with an objective account of what has happened.

When you speak to the consultant radiologist supervising you, they remark that 'a patient of her age shouldn't have got pregnant in the first place'.

GMC Good Medical Practice states that 'you must not unfairly discriminate against patients or colleagues by allowing your personal views to affect the treatment you provide or arrange'. Although this may be an isolated comment it certainly raises questions about your colleague's integrity. If there is concern you should escalate the event to your educational supervisor.

Summary

Radiologists are obliged to protect patients from the harmful effects of exposure to ionising radiation and to weigh up the risks and benefits of any scan. Departmental procedures are in place to aid this process. Any breach in regulation should be appropriately escalated and the patient fully counselled on the relevant adverse effects.

> **TOP TIPS**
>
> ✚ Familiarise yourself with IRMER procedures in practice in your local radiology department. Do not deny a patient the right to complain, even if it is about you.
>
> ✚ Documentation is key.

5.2.4 Confidentiality

Scenario

You are the ST1 radiology trainee about to present your audit at the departmental audit meeting. You saved patient images on an unencrypted memory stick which you realise you have misplaced somewhere in the hospital. What do you do?

Questions

How would you approach this scenario?

Seek information: You will need to consider when you last had the memory stick and where in the hospital you have been with it since. Was the data anonymised? Had the patient consented to your use of the images?

Patient safety: Although there is no immediate risk to patient safety this serious breach of information governance guidelines puts the patient's confidentiality at risk. A breach in confidentiality will adversely affect a patient's trust in the hospital and therefore their future interactions with the healthcare profession.

Initiative: This incident is more important than your presentation at a departmental meeting and you will need to take steps to look for the memory stick as soon as possible. You should start by contacting the meeting chair to explain why you cannot attend.

Escalate: The severity of this situation should not be underestimated, you will need to escalate to your educational supervisor immediately. The situation will likely then be escalated to the departmental head and the trust's Caldicott guardian. An incident form should also be completed.

Support: The patient should be notified about what has happened and be offered an apology. They should also be kept up-to-date about the investigation into the incident and measures taken to prevent such an incident happening again.

What are the key issues?

This station tests your knowledge of the Data Protection Act (1998) as well as information governance and confidentiality issues. These concepts are not specific to radiology and so you should be familiar with the relevant guidelines. Furthermore, in this situation you are asked how you would deal with realising you have done something wrong, thereby testing your integrity.

Are you aware of any guidelines relating to the use of memory sticks?

Memory sticks should not be used for long-term storage of information and should only be used as a means for transportation of information from one location to another. Most trusts have local guidelines which state that if personal information is to be transferred to a memory stick it must be via a trust-approved encrypted device which may be obtained from the local IT department or equivalent. Unencrypted memory sticks should never be used for personal identifiable information.

On explaining the situation to the patient in question they ask what will happen next

You should explain that an incident form will be completed and that the incident will be escalated to the head of department as well as the trust Caldicott guardian. These measures will result in a full investigation into the incident, the outcome of which will guide steps to prevent a similar event happening in the future. The patient may also ask about procedures to lodge a complaint, in this instance information about the local Patient Advice and Liaison Services should be provided.

What does the Caldicott guardian do?

The Caldicott guardian is a senior trust employee who is responsible for protecting patient confidentiality and overseeing the appropriate sharing of patient information.

What are the possible repercussions of this event?

Depending on the nature of the information lost the incident may be escalated to the Senior Information Risk Owner (SIRO) of the hospital or even further to the Information Commissioner (ICO). The patient would also have the right to take legal action, as their information has not been protected. Outcomes may include a financial penalty for the hospital as well as disciplinary action for you including information governance training and a verbal or written warning.

You recall that you may have taken the memory stick to the canteen earlier that day, however, when you return to look the canteen is locked as lunchtime is over

There should be no delay looking for the memory stick; you cannot risk someone else finding the memory stick if there is a chance it is still in the canteen. In this scenario, you should contact hospital security, explain what has happened and ask for access into the canteen to look.

You confide in a colleague about what has happened and they encourage you to ignore the incident as whoever finds the memory stick is unlikely to be able to interpret the images anyway

You cannot make assumptions about who will have access to the lost information. Ignoring the incident may have worse repercussions for you in the long term as it may appear as though you were trying to cover up what has happened. This would call into question your probity and would be reason for GMC involvement. It will be far more favourable for you to own up to what has happened at the earliest opportunity.

Summary

Patients have a right to confidentiality and there is a legal obligation to handle confidential information securely. If memory sticks are used to transfer patient identifiable information they should be trust approved and encrypted. Breaches in information security are taken very seriously.

TOP TIPS

 Review your local information governance guidelines; ignorance of local protocol is not a defence.

5.2.5 Radiation protection incident

Scenario
You are the junior registrar reporting CT. The radiographer informs you that a 32-year-old man referred for an ultrasound has mistakenly had a CT instead. How do you proceed?

Questions
How would you approach this scenario?

Seek information: Importantly you need to assess the exact nature of the case. Gather information on how this mistake has arisen. Were the correct ID checks carried out? Is there a patient in the hospital who was meant to have the CT instead? Is the patient aware of the mistake yet?

Patient safety: There is generally no immediate threat to patient safety, but there are potential long term complications of ionising radiation. More important short term risks include potential contrast allergies and contrast-induced renal injury. Assess the patient and their history for either of these possibilities. It is important to document what has happened clearly in the patient notes if possible.

Initiative: Explain to the patient clearly that there has been a mistake, ensuring apologies are made and measures will be taken to prevent future occurrences. An incident form should also be completed.

Escalate: Ensure you discuss the incident with the RPS (usually a senior radiographer) so that appropriate measures are taken to document and learn from this mistake. The RPA should also be informed to calculate the radiation dose and counsel the patient regarding the risks of their exposure. You would likely discuss with the consultant running the CT list who could support you in dealing with this incident.

Support: This situation tests your probity and communication skills in dealing with a serious incident. It is important that despite the wrong investigation being performed, it should be reported in a timely manner and may still assist in making a diagnosis. Should an ultrasound still be required, this should be arranged without further delay.

What are the key issues?

The main issues involve clear communication and honesty. Once a radiation protection incident has occurred, it is your responsibility to communicate with the patient honestly, ensure the scan is reported in a timely manner and escalate to the appropriate people. This will ensure that right measures are taken to prevent a future incident from occurring.

The Old Interview Stations: 5.2.5 Radiation Protection Incident

The patient asks if there are any risks to the CT scan?

Ionising radiation is a form of electromagnetic radiation that can cause structural damage to DNA. The risk to a patient comes from the dose of radiation absorbed and the length of time post-radiation. There are two categories of effect: deterministic effects (which are dose-dependent) and stochastic effects (unrelated to dose) such as malignancy. If a patient asks then you must not lie about these effects and it would be a case of gauging their current level of understanding and determining how much information they would like to know. It may not be appropriate in the first instance to unsettle a patient about the risk of future malignancy with a 40-year lag period. It would be more appropriate to reassure the patient that diagnostic dose levels are generally safe unless a dose limit has been exceeded. You could advise them that if they remain concerned you will put them in touch with the medical physics department at the earliest opportunity. You can also advise the patient that if they wish to make a formal complaint of how to do so (e.g. Patient Advice and Liaison Services), but where possible it is better to resolve issues informally at the time.

Summary

This scenario is a test of honesty, clear communication and appropriate escalation. It is important to understand some of the risks of ionising radiation (stochastic versus non-stochastic) and be aware of radiation protection legislation including IRMER. Importantly, in this case the issues are regarding an inappropriate scan and trying to learn from a mistake. The scenario would change slightly if the issue was a dose of radiation much greater than intended, whether due to faulty equipment or human error. This would follow slightly different procedures and understanding of the deterministic effects (including skin necrosis) become more important.

TOP TIPS

✚ Gather information regarding the nature of the mistake and ensure clear communication with senior colleagues, the RPS/RPA and most of all the patient affected.

✚ Gauge the level of information to give to the patient, reassure the patient, explain the steps that will be taken in the future to prevent this issue from happening again and how they can get in touch if they feel necessary at a later date. Explain that the scan may still be useful and could find a diagnosis that an ultrasound may not have seen.

5.2.6 Contrast reaction

Scenario
During a busy senior registrar on-call, the radiographer phones to tell you that an 8-year-old girl has just come out of the CT scanner looking unwell and sounding wheezy. How do you proceed?

Questions
How would you approach this scenario?

Seek information: This scenario is a potential medical emergency as a child that is unwell and wheezy may be having an acute reaction to the contrast medium. You must safely but quickly proceed to the CT scanning room. Whilst on the phone you may wish to ask the radiographer to get the contrast reaction/crash trolley.

Patient Safety: This is paramount. You are dealing with a potentially acutely unwell child and time is of the essence.

Initiative: You must be able to perform an ABCDE assessment of the patient.

Escalate: If possible inform the consultant running the CT list or ask a colleague to do so. If in any doubt regarding the well-being of the child an arrest call should be put out (2222 in acute UK hospitals) which ensures additional help is obtained. In any case, you are likely to want to inform the paediatric registrar of what is happening.

Support: Utilise other colleagues in these scenarios to help in what can be a stressful environment. It is important to act calmly to minimise mistakes. There will be worried parents in the room and dealing with them can be challenging.

What are the key issues?

Patient safety is paramount. You should have adequate knowledge of how to manage a contrast reaction. It is important to recognise a clinically deteriorating patient and escalate appropriately. It is also important to document clearly in the notes the timeline of events. Finally, good communication is essential with a likely worried child who may be confused and frightened. It is also important to communicate clearly with the parents what is happening.

How do you manage a contrast reaction?

Treatment ranges from supportive with observation to active medical management. It is important to assess the range of contrast reactions, from urticaria and nausea, to laryngospasm/laryngeal oedema and full anaphylaxis. If there is evidence of laryngospasm then high flow oxygen/beta agonists can be given. At interview, you may be asked the emergency management of anaphylaxis particularly as this is the most life-threatening. It is important to advise you will manage in a logical ABCDE approach. This would include calling the crash team, suctioning the airway if needed, elevating the patient's legs if hypotensive, oxygen (6-10 l/min), adrenaline 1:1000 0.3ml (0.3mg) IM (do not confuse dose with management of PEA/asystolic cardiac arrest which uses 1:10000 IV adrenaline). You may also use other adjuvants such as antihistamines (for example chlorphenamine 5 mg IM/IV), steroids or bronchodilators. Doses given are for an 8-year-old child, but you should mention that you would check the BNF for children for accurate doses. Also refer to the Resuscitation Council (UK) guidelines.

The parents are terribly anxious and are panicking about their child, what do you do?

The safety of the child is paramount in this situation. It is more important to provide treatment to stabilise the child than discuss with the parents in the acute stage. In practice these things tend to occur simultaneously depending on the number of people present. If the child is well enough you may have time to explain, but most likely a colleague will discuss with the parents in a separate room. If the crash team are managing the patient, then it may be up to you as a radiology registrar to communicate effectively what is happening. Clearly explain what has happened and what the medical team are doing to help the situation.

Summary

The issues are: patient safety, knowledge of the range of contrast reactions, how to deal with contrast reactions clinically, clear documentation and clear communication with the patient and parents. Contrast reactions are uncommon but it is vital for a radiologist to know how to treat these reactions in a safe and timely manner. It is important to make it clear that escalation would be appropriate particularly involving the hospital crash team and paediatric registrar.

TOP TIPS

✚ Logical assessment of the patient using an ABCDE approach

✚ Clear communication and demonstrate an ability to lead an emergency scenario including delegation of roles *(such as asking a radiographer to cannulate, or escort parents).*

✚ Knowledge of medical management of anaphylaxis including drug doses.

✚ Ensuring patient safety is paramount including timely and appropriate escalation and calling the crash team without hesitation.

5.2.7 Jehovah's witness

Scenario

You are the ST6 interventional radiologist on-call. You are about to perform a coil embolisation on a patient who has presented to A&E with an acute GI bleed. You would like to arrange for a blood transfusion, however the accompanying relatives tell you that the patient is a Jehovah's Witness. What would you do?

Questions
How would you approach this scenario?

Seek information: It will be important to discuss this with the patient if possible (he or she may not be competent). For example, what would the patient find acceptable in terms of blood products or "bloodless" products? Discussing with the family will also be important - ultimately, you may need to act in the patient's best interests and the family will help you determine what these are. Is there disagreement amongst relatives? In which case, you may err more towards the side of giving the transfusion. Try and find out what alternative options there are e.g. Can it be done without a blood transfusion? Can it be delayed until more information is gathered? Are there any blood-free alternatives?

Other information:
 • Is there a valid advanced directive?
 • Other evidence of valid refusal e.g. documentation in the notes?
 • Does the patient have a legal representative?

Patient Safety: Bear in mind that ultimately your duty is to the patient's best interests and their safety. If the patient is not competent and the situation becomes life-threatening, it may be the right decision to arrange a blood transfusion against the relatives' wishes. Remember that legally, if the patient lacks capacity, relatives and others only have an advisory role, although consensus amongst all involved parties is advised.

Initiative: Part of taking initiative will be to escalate such a complex situation early; you would not be expected to deal with this problem alone (see below). The course of action will change significantly depending on the patient's capacity. If the patient has capacity, then you must respect their decision, even if it seems irrational. If you are unsure of their capacity to consent, then a senior opinion is particularly important, as well as potentially that of a psychiatrist. If the patient does not have capacity, then determine if the lack of capacity is temporary or permanent. Consult the family and rest of your team to determine the patient's best interests. It may be necessary to begin the steps towards seeking a court order (time allowing).

Other practical steps would include stabilising the patient as much as possible (e.g. fluid resuscitation if appropriate, appropriate level of care) and preparing in case the final decision is to go ahead with the transfusion and procedure i.e. blood available and interventional suite/staff ready.

Escalate: Involve your consultant, even if this means waking them up in the night. It may be necessary to even involve a person of higher responsibility e.g. the medical director, as there may be legal issues. Other people to consider seeking advice from include: an advocate for Jehovah's witnesses (The Watchtower society, the governing body of the Jehovah's Witness) and any available ethical/legal liaison (via hospital or medical defence union).

Support: This sort of situation can be difficult and stressful for all parties involved. Offer support to other members of your team and seek support for yourself, if necessary.

What are the key issues?

Ethical principles of beneficence, non-maleficence and autonomy. Remember autonomy takes precedence over both beneficence and non-maleficence, if the patient is competent. Competence = a patient's capacity to make medical decisions. As per the Mental Capacity Act 2005, to demonstrate capacity, a patient must:
- Understand the information provided in relation to the decision
- Retain the information
- Use and weigh up that information
- Communicate their decision, by whatever means possible

What if you cannot get hold of your on-call consultant?

Consider contacting another consultant (e.g. the clinical director of your department). Failing that, consider involving a consultant from another involved specialty (e.g. medical, surgical or ITU). You may be forced to escalate to the medical director. If really forced to make a decision, ensure that you have legal advice (e.g. medical defence union) and that you have documented all discussions and the entire decision process. Bear in mind, it may be easier to defend keeping the patient alive, rather than letting the patient die.

What if the patient is a child and the parents are refusing a blood transfusion on his behalf?

Depending on the age of the patient, you may have to apply the principles of Gillick competence. The guidelines are that in an emergency, you can treat a child without consent however consensus with the parents is, of course, preferred. This will again involve discussions regarding alternative products and treatment options. Senior involvement and legal advice remain vital.

Summary

This is an extremely challenging scenario for which there isn't really a correct answer. There are multiple ethical and legal principles which can be covered and you should be familiar with all of these, should the interviewers decide to stop and probe further. Essentially, the discussion you have with the interviewers will be determined by whether the patient is competent or not. Likely, the interviewer will want to lead you down the path of no competence in order to test your knowledge of competence/capacity and assessment of best interests.

TOP TIPS

 Don't commit yourself to 'transfusion' or 'no transfusion' early on. Take the time to discuss the possibilities.

5.2.8 Inappropriate referral

Scenario

You are the junior registrar on-call. The vascular surgery consultant calls saying his wife has a chronic headache and would like a CT head scan. How do you respond?

Questions
How would you approach this scenario?

Seek information: The vascular consultant will obviously be concerned about his wife's wellbeing. Seek information in a sensitive manner, without specifically refusing to do the scan. Find out the full clinical picture. How urgently does the scan need to be performed? Can it wait for a discussion with your own senior? What is your current workload? There are likely to be other scans waiting that are more clinically urgent.

Patient Safety: Your duty remains with the patient, who in this case is the vascular consultant's wife. If you believe she requires urgent imaging you should advise a more appropriate pathway, which would be through A&E (who would then request the scan and follow it up).

Initiative: The bottom line here is that it is an inappropriate referral pathway. But, as with all referrals, it should be dealt with in a professional manner. Discuss the case as you would any other and come to your own opinion regarding its appropriateness and clinical urgency. Part of your role within IRMER is to justify the radiation dose. Consider whether this is the correct modality – from the basic information provided (chronic headache), MRI may in fact provide more information and avoid an unnecessary dose of radiation. Explaining this to the vascular consultant may in fact allow you to come to a compromise. You still, however, shouldn't agree to a MRI scan without an appropriate referral pathway.

Escalate: Do not feel coerced into vetting a scan which you do not feel is appropriate, even if it is coming from a consultant clinician. If necessary, involve your own consultant. It may be appropriate for your consultant to discuss this with the vascular consultant directly.

Support: Although you may disagree on the correct management, you should empathise with the vascular consultant, who will obviously be worried about his wife.

What are the key issues?

The keys issues involve having an understanding of appropriate referral pathways and appreciating professional boundaries, whilst demonstrating understanding towards another colleague's concerns.
You should demonstrate your clinical acumen, in terms of being aware of potentially more appropriate imaging modalities.

What if the vascular consultant becomes aggressive or rude and insists on getting a CT scan?

You should deal with this professionally and politely, but explain your reasoning and ultimately, stand your ground. Remember your duty is to the patient, and you should not perform a CT scan which you do not feel can be justified (review the role of a radiologist within IRMER). If you feel you have been treated inappropriately, you should escalate this to your consultant on-call the following day.

Is a CT scan ever indicated in a chronic headache?

This is a difficult question to answer without more specifics about the patient's signs and symptoms
For example, it may still be appropriate to rule out a space occupying lesion using CT in the first instance. This decision will also depend on other factors such as the patient's age (consideration given to radiation) and availability of the two modalities (MRI may not be available out of hours).

Summary

The referral pathway is inappropriate but it still warrants a fair discussion as with any other request. Determine the full clinical picture before coming to a final decision and ask your questions sensitively as the vascular consultant will be concerned about his wife. Determine if this scan is indicated, the urgency of it and whether the this is the correct modality. If you feel it isn't, explain your reasoning and offer an alternative plan. Do not be afraid to involve your senior if necessary.

Printed in Great Britain
by Amazon